Beyond the natural I

MW00334402

Beyond the Natural Body presents an episode in the history of life sciences that is essential to our current understanding of sex and the body, and the relations between gender and science. Since the early decades of the twentieth century, the notion of the hormonally constructed body has become the dominant mode of conceptualizing bodies, particularly female bodies, to such an extent that we now assume that it is a natural phenomenon. This book challenges the idea that there is such a thing as a "natural" body and demonstrates that it is the process by which scientific claims achieve universal status that constructs such discourses as natural facts.

Beyond the Natural Body tells the fascinating story of scientists' search for the many tons of ovaries, testes and urine that were required in experiments to develop the hormonal body concept. It traces the origins of sex hormones and follows their development through mass-production as drugs to their eventual transformation into the contraceptive pill. Nelly Oudshoorn argues that the power to control sex and the body is not restricted to the domain of texts and ideologies. In addition, she describes the dynamic, capillary action of a science which linked cultural assumptions, concepts, ovaries, urine, diagnostic tests, laboratory equipment, marketing strategies, clinical trials, population policies and bodies, thus transforming the world we live in.

Nelly Oudshoorn is Assistant Professor in the Department of Science Dynamics at the University of Amsterdam, and has written numerous articles on gender and biology.

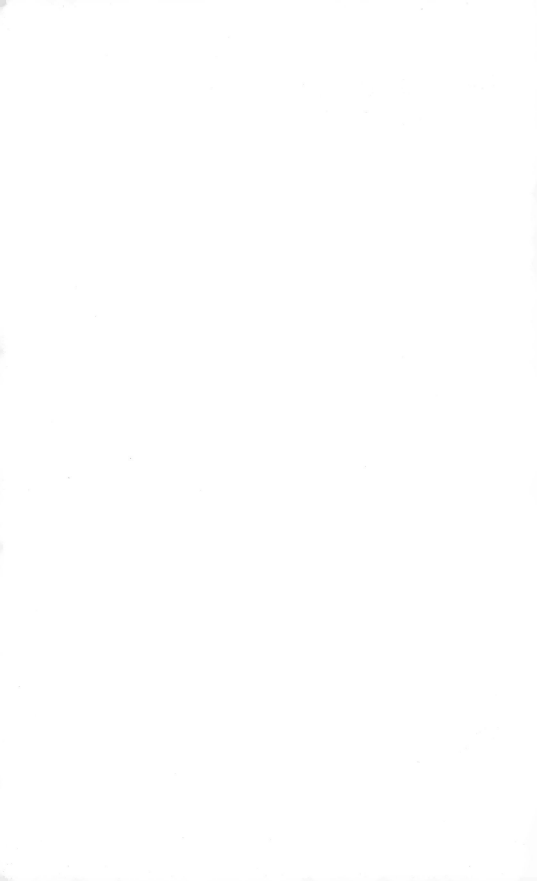

Beyond the natural body

An archeology of sex hormones

Nelly Oudshoorn

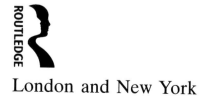

London and New York

First published 1994
by Routledge
11 New Fetter Lane, London EC4P 4EE

Simultaneously published in the USA and Canada
by Routledge
29 West 35th Street, New York, NY 10001

Phototypeset in Times by Intype, London
Printed and bound in Great Britain by
Biddles Ltd, Guildford and King's Lynn

British Library Cataloguing in Publication Data
A catalogue record for this book is available from the British Library.

Library of Congress Cataloging in Publication Data
Oudshoorn, Nelly, 1950–
  Beyond the natural body : an archeology of sex hormones / Nelly
Oudshoorn.
  p.   cm.
  Includes bibliographical references and index.
  1. Sex hormones—Research—History—20th century. I. Title.
QP572.S4083 1994
612.6—dc20   94–4945

ISBN 0–415–09190-X (hbk)
ISBN 0–415–09191–8 (pbk)

For Maartje and Rob

Contents

Figures

Preface and acknowledgements

In the early 1980s, my feminist friends repeatedly asked me to explain what biologists have had to say about women, and why it is that women are depicted as determined and limited by their "biological nature" in ways that men, in general, are not. Despite my years of education in biology, I had no answers to their questions. These questions led me and other biology students to found the women's group in biology. The very first ideas for this book stem from the many evenings of discussions I shared with this group. The subject of women's biology turned out to be profoundly political, and was at that time not yet subjected to any systemic feminist inquiry. We discussed our objections to the determinism and reductionism of biological theories relating to sex differences, and the implications of such theories for feminism. The women's group proved to be a very creative and productive context for developing ideas and strategies to introduce the subject of women and biology to the agenda of the university curriculum. Thanks to the efforts of this group, this issue became institutionalized as a new field in women's studies at the University of Amsterdam. The major part of the work presented in this book was done in the socially and intellectually stimulating atmosphere surrounding the establishment of this new research field.

There are, inevitably, a great many people whose ideas, inspiration and support have contributed to the realization of this book: Olga Amsterdamska, Louis Boon, Teresa Brennan, Christien Brouwer, Adele Clarke, Jacqueline Cramer, Diana Long, Annemarie Mol, Nanne van der Poll, Koos Slob, Anne Fausto Sterling, Marianne van den Wijngaard, and Ineke van Wingerden. I am grateful for the help of all these colleagues and friends who have provided me with the knowledge, skills and energy that made the writing of this book into such an intellectually exciting endeavor.

My work has been greatly facilitated by the cooperation of the – unfortunately now late – Professor Dr Marius Tausk, and of Dr. Ina Uyldert, who gave detailed accounts of their experiences in the field of sex hormones in the 1920s and 1930s. I gratefully acknowledge the permission of Dr. K. Wiedhaup to consult the Organon Archives containing the correspondence of Professor Dr. Ernst Laqueur, and the assistance of the library staff of the Faculty of Biology at the University of Amsterdam in collecting the relevant literature on sex hormones. I wish to thank Gene Moore in particular for his skillful and thorough editing of the translations.

Last, but not least, I would like to express my gratitude to my family and friends. To my parents for providing me with the opportunity to complete a higher education, which enabled me to leave my job in a small town pharmacy for a then unknown but exciting future. To my friend Rob Vrakking for providing me with the ideal condition for the birth of this book: a creative silence.

Some of these chapters are based on previously published materials. Chapter 2 was first published in the *Journal of the History of Biology*, 1990, 23 (2): 163–186; an earlier version of Chapter 3 appeared in *Bulletin of the History of Medicine* 1990, 64: 243–261; Chapter 4 has been published in *Social Studies of Science* 1990, 20: 5–33; and a shorter version of Chapter 5 appeared in *Science, Technology and Human Values*, 1993, 18: 5–25.

I gratefully acknowledge the permission of AKZO, Organon International BV, to use the photographs of the early laboratory work on sex hormones (Chapters 3, 4 and 5) and *Chemisch Weekblad*, *The Lancet* and *Nature* for permission to use the photographs of publications on sex hormones (Chapters 2 and 5).

However natural categories are, we need to search whether and by what means they find their existence as natural categories.

(Coupland 1988)

Bodies are not born, they are made.

(Haraway 1989b: 10)

1 Introduction

"When you meet a human being," Freud has said, "the first distinction you make is 'male or female', and you are accustomed to making the distinction with unhesitating certainty," (Freud 1933: 120 as cited in Strachney 1965). In the early decades of the twentieth century, scientists were less confident about the distinctions between female and male characteristics:

> Although the classification into male and female sex hormones seems self-evident, it is nevertheless rather difficult to define; the changing opinions hereabout have succeeded one another so fast in such a small number of years, that at present it looks like chaos. . . . The major problem is that precise notions associated with the words male and female are, alas, merely the property of the laymen, and fade away more and more if one becomes acquainted with the progressing experimental-biological research. We find it increasingly difficult to define which observed characteristics can be considered decisive for our judgement: male or female.
>
> (Jongh 1936: 5, 306)

Beyond the Natural Body focuses on this episode in the 1920s and 1930s in which scientists became confused by their own assumptions about sex and the body.

UNDER THE SPELL OF THE BODY

What about sex and the body? Early-twentieth-century scientists were definitely not the only ones who struggled with the question of how we can think about female and male bodies. During the second wave of feminism that started in the 1970s, (fe)male bodies were of central concern in many debates, although in a rather peculiar way. Feminist biologists, like myself, were certain that biological determinism had to be rejected. We knew that nature does not determine what we mean when we use terms such as woman, body, femininity. We chose this position to contest those opponents of feminism who suggested that social inequality between women and men is primarily rooted in biological sex differences. According to this opinion, social changes demanded by feminists are wishful thinking because biology, rather than society, sets constraints on the behavior and abilities of women. Biology is destiny, and feminists simply have to accept this reality.

At this juncture in history, we could have chosen to question this "reality," particularly the assumption that there exists such a thing as a natural body. We might have questioned the status of the biomedical sciences as providers of objective truth, and their assumed role of objective arbiters in social debates. Whatever else may have happened in these exciting years, feminists did not take up this challenge. The biomedical sciences were not included in the feminist research agenda.

Instead we focused our attention on the social sciences. Simone de Beauvoir's argument that "women are made, not born" functioned as a paradigm for feminist scholars in sociology, anthropology, and psychology seeking to analyze the social and cultural contexts of sexual inequality.[1] In the course of the 1970s, feminists introduced the concept of gender – as distinct from sex – into the discourse on women. In *Sex, Gender and Society* (1972), the British sociologist Ann Oakley emphasized the relevance of making a distinction between "biological, innate sex differences" and "gender attributes that are acquired by socialization."[2] In 1975, the American anthropologist Gayle Rubin extended the concept of gender from sociology to anthropology. Rubin included the concept of gender in her influential theory of the sex–gender system to describe the cultural and social structures in which women become excluded from tasks and qualities considered as masculine (Rubin 1975). In this approach, the use of the concept of sex became restricted to biological sex, implicitly or explicitly specified in terms of anatomical, hormonal or chromosomal criteria. Gender is used to refer to all other "socially constructed characteristics" attributed to women and men, such as specific psychological and behavioral characteristics, social roles, and particular types of jobs.

What actually happened was that feminists, by introducing the sex–gender distinction, reproduced the traditional task division between the social sciences and the biomedical sciences. Feminists assigned the study of sex to the domain of the biomedical sciences, and defined the study of gender as the exclusive domain of the social sciences.[3] My point here is not to deny the productivity of the introduction of the sex–gender distinction. The 1970s witnessed the publication of numerous gender studies that revealed the social, cultural, and psychological conditions in which girls and women acquire a feminine role and identity. My argument is that the sex–gender distinction did not challenge the notion of a natural body. Although the concept of gender was developed to contest the naturalization of femininity, the opposite has happened. Feminist theories of socialization did not question the biological sex of those subjects that become socialized as woman; they took sex and the body for granted as unchanging biological realities that needed no further explanation (Duden 1991c: vi,vii,3; Moll 1988). In these studies, the concept of sex maintained its status as an ahistorical attribute of the human body and the body remained excluded from feminist analysis.

It was in the late 1970s and early 1980s that the body made its first appearance in feminist writings. Historians proposed to include the female body in feminist research. In "La Storia delle Donna", Gianna Pomata challenged the assumption that the female body has a universal, transhistorical essence (Pomata 1983). In the tradition of Pomata, women's history now focused on the particular historicity of women's experiences with their bodies. These studies showed most powerfully how our perceptions of the female body are always subject to historical change. "We cannot speak of the female body as if it were an invariant presence through history. There is no fixed, experiental base which provides continuity across the centuries" (Jacobus *et al.* 1990: 4).

In addition to historians, anthropologists also came under the spell of the body. Anthropologists brought the awareness that perceptions of one's body are bound by culture and stressed the cross-cultural diversity of bodily experiences. Each culture attributes different meanings to the female body. Emily Martin's book *The Woman in the Body* extended the anthropological approach to the experiences of women in contemporary American culture. Martin showed how women's imaging of their bodies vary even within one culture, due to differences in social and economic backgrounds (Martin 1987).

Anthropologists and historians provided very powerful insights that challenged the notion of a natural body. However, they went only halfway. These studies focused on experiences with the body and on how these experiences are molded by time and culture. This still leaves room for the argument that, despite differences in bodily experiences, these experiences do refer to a universal, physiological reality, "a non-historical biological matter" (Duden 1991c: 6). In the experiental approach the facticity and self-evidence of "biological facts" about the body remained unchallenged.[4]

Feminist biologists and historians of science did not hesitate to make this crucial move in exposing the myth of the natural body. Ruth Bleier, Ruth Hubbard, Evelyn Fox Keller and Helen Longino suggested that anatomical, endocrinological or immunological "facts" are anything but self-evident.[5] From these feminist scholars I adopted the intellectually challenging and politically relevant notion that there does not exist an unmediated natural truth of the body. Our perceptions and interpretations of the body are mediated through language and, in our society, the biomedical sciences function as a major provider of this language.[6] This view of the body is linked to a critical reappraisal of the status of biomedical knowledge. If understanding the body is mediated by language, scientists are bound by language as well. Consequently, the assumption that the biomedical sciences are the providers of objective knowledge about the "true nature" of the body could be rejected. This really changed my view of science and the world. What is science all about if scientists are not discovering reality? In search of an answer to this question I was inspired by the literature of the emerging field of social studies of science that introduced the powerful idea that scientific facts are not objectively given, but collectively created.[7] This implies a totally different perspective on what scientists are doing: scientists are actively constructing reality, rather than discovering reality. For the debate about the body, this means that the naturalistic reality of the body as such does not exist, it is created by scientists as the object of scientific investigation (Duden 1991c: 22). The social constructivist approach opened up a whole new line of research exposing the multiple ways in which the biomedical sciences as discursive technologies (re)construct and reflect our understanding of the body.[8] The body, in all its complexities, thus achieved an important position on the feminist research agenda.

Studies since the early 1980s provide a fascinating view of the richness and complexity of biomedical discourses concerning the body through the centuries. One of the most conspicuous ideas emerging from these studies is that the biomedical sciences have led to a fragmentation of the body. However contradictory it may seem, the body as a unity, the object of biomedical research *par excellence*, gradually disappeared from biomedical discourse. The practices of eighteenth-century anatomy transformed the body into detachable pieces. Medical men dissected the body into smaller units that were subsequently renamed and classified. These "organs without bodies," to use the words of Rosi Braidotti, came to replace the body as a unity (Braidotti 1989). Since the late nineteenth century, medical research has gone well beyond the organs. Research in histology, molecular biology, biochemistry, endocrinology and neurobiology focuses on tissues, cells, micro-organisms, hormones and neurotransmitters (Braidotti 1991: 362). Thanks to transplantation science and reproductive technologies parts of our bodies can now be transferred from person to person. Hearts, kidneys, eyes, tissues, eggs, sperm and embryos are moved from body to body (Martin 1987).

Another thread that runs through the history of the biomedical sciences is their power to visualize the "secrets" of the body. Modern science made the invisible visible. The dissection practices of eighteenth-century anatomy literally opened the body to the scrutiny of medical scientists and shifted the medical gaze from the superficial contours of the body to its insides (Braidotti 1991: 361; T. Laqueur 1990). Anatomy opened up new, unexplored spaces in the body. Modern visualization techniques have further extended this tradition and enabled medical scientists to penetrate into places that remained hidden to their colleagues in earlier centuries. Nineteenth-century X-rays made visible parts of the body that could not be studied with the dissection techniques of anatomists: chests and lungs in motion, in bodies that were still alive (Pasveer 1992). Since the mid-twentieth century, ultra-sound technologies have made possible the visualization of every imaginable part of the body, depicting even the fetus in the womb (Blume 1992; Duden 1991b).

With the rise of modern science, bodies have thus become transformed into objects that can be manipulated with an ever growing number of tools and techniques. Bodies in biomedical discourse are "useful, purposeful bodies that can produce knowledge" (Braidotti 1991: 361). Medical technologies have transformed our understanding of "the natural body." Biomedical discourses, however, not only are shaped by technological developments, but also shift in response to changes in society. The very words used to capture the complexities of the body show a changing set of metaphors that reflect the values of a specific historical period: bodies in scientific texts are "woven from the same materials of the social imagination that go into the making of a new society" (Duden 1991c: 26). Medical men seem to have been particularly prone to describe bodily processes in terms of economical modes of thinking. Metaphors reflecting the specific economical organizations of society are abundant in medical representations of the body. In the nineteenth century, for instance, the body was described as a small business trying to spend, save or balance its accounts, thus mirroring the values of early capitalism. Spending-saving metaphors dominated the description of physiological processes and diseases. Processes in the cell were, for instance, described as processes of income and expenditure that must be kept in balance (Martin 1987: 32). In the early twentieth century the body came to be represented as a model of an industrial society, with the cell as a factory (Martin 1987: 36–37). In the 1950s, bodies became complex technological communication systems, an imagery of the body that is still dominant in the 1990s. Fields such as endocrinology, immunology and the neurosciences described bodily processes in terms of complicated communication systems between organs and entities such as hormones and neurotransmitters (Haraway 1989b: 16). Most importantly, the use of metaphors is not just a game with words. Metaphors entail specific meanings and values that may contribute to a positive or negative attitude toward the body. The representation of menstruation in terms of failed production, for instance, seems to facilitate a rather negative view of it (Martin 1987: 45).

In summary, feminist studies of the biomedical sciences have shown us how at crucial points medical technologies have shaped what we consider as our bodies.[9] The technology of childbirth has fundamentally shifted our understanding of birth itself: the role of the mother has been written out of the process of birth which is transformed into an interaction between doctor and fetus (Treichler 1990). Contraceptive technologies have revolutionized sexual experiences, separating sexuality from reproduction, whereas in vitro fertilization techniques have drastically changed our perceptions of motherhood by introducing categories such as "gestational mother" and "genetic mother."

SEX AND THE BODY

In these biomedical discourses, the construction of the body as something with a sex has been a central theme all through the centuries. The myriad ways in which scientists have understood sex provide many illuminating counter-moves to the argument that sex is an unequivocal, ahistorical attribute of the body that, once unveiled by science, is valid everywhere and within every context. Early medical texts in particular challenge our present-day perceptions of male and female bodies. For our postmodern minds it is hard to imagine that for two thousand years, male and female bodies were not conceptualized in terms of differences. Medical texts from the ancient Greeks until the late eighteenth century described male and female bodies as fundamentally similar. Women had even the same genitals as men, with one difference: "theirs are inside the body and not outside it." In this approach, characterized by Thomas Laqueur as the "one-sex model," the female body was understood as a "male turned inside herself," not a different sex, but a lesser version of the male body (T. Laqueur 1990). Medical textbooks of this period show drawings of the female genitals that stress their resemblance to male genitalia so vividly that one could believe them to be representations of the male penis. For thousands of years the "one-sex model" dominated biomedical discourse, even to such an extent that medical texts lacked a specific anatomical nomenclature for female reproductive organs. The ovary, for instance did not have a name of its own, but was described as the female testicle, thus referring again to the male organ. The language we are now familiar with, such as vagina and clitoris, simply did not exist (T. Laqueur 1990: 5,96).

This emphasis on similarities rather than differences is also present in the texts of anatomists who studied parts of the body other than the reproductive organs. For Vesalius, the father of anatomy, "sex was only skin deep, limited to differences in the outline of the body and the organs of reproduction. In his view, all other organs were interchangeable between the sexes" (Schiebinger 1989: 189). In his beautiful drawings of the skeleton in *Epitome*, an anatomical atlas that appeared in 1543, Vesalius did not give a sex to the bony structure of the body (Schiebinger 1989: 182). This (as we would now perceive it) "indifference" of medical scientists to bodily differences between the sexes does not seem to be a consequence of ignorance of the female body. Since the fourteenth century, the dissection of women's bodies was part of anatomical practice (Schiebinger 1989: 182). According to Laqueur, the stress on similarities, representing the female body as just a gradation of one basic male type, was inextricably intertwined with patriarchal thinking, reflecting the values of an overwhelmingly male public world in which "man is the measure of all things, and woman does not exist as an ontologically distinct category" (T. Laqueur 1990: 62).

It was only in the eighteenth century that biomedical discourse first included a concept of sex that is more familiar to our present-day interpretations of the male and the female body. The long established tradition that emphasized bodily similarities over differences began to be heavily criticized. In the mid-eighteenth century, anatomists increasingly focused on bodily differences between the sexes, and argued that sex was not restricted to the reproductive organs, or as one physician put it: "the essence of sex is not confined to a single organ but extends, through more or less perceptible nuances, into every part" (Schiebinger 1989: 189). The first part of the body to become sexualized was the skeleton. If sex differences could be found in "the hardest part of the body," it would be likely that sex penetrated "every muscle, vein, and organ attached to and molded by the skeleton" (Schiebinger 1989: 191). In the 1750s, the first female skeletons appeared in medical textbooks. Londa Schiebinger has described how anatomists paid special attention to those parts of the skeleton that would become socially significant, amongst which was the skull. The depiction of the female skull was used to prove that women's intellectual capacities were inferior to those of men (Schiebinger 1986). The history of medicine in this period contains many illustrations of similar reflections of the social role of women in the representation of the human body. Anatomists of more recent centuries "mended nature to fit emerging ideals of masculinity and femininity" (Schiebinger 1989: 203).[10] In nineteenth-century cellular physiology the medical gaze shifted from the bones to the cells. Physiological "facts" were used to explain the passive nature of women. The biomedical sciences thus functioned as an arbiter in socio-political debates about women's rights and abilities (T. Laqueur 1990: 6, 215).

By the late nineteenth century medical scientists had extended this sexualization to every imaginable part of the body: bones, blood vessels, cells, hair and brains (Schiebinger 1989: 189). Only the eye seems to have no sex (Honegger 1991: 176). Biomedical discourse thus shows a clear shift in focus from similarities to differences.[11] The female and the male body now became conceptualized in terms of opposite bodies with "incommensurably different organs, functions, and feelings" (T. Laqueur 1990: viii).

Following this shift, the female body became the medical object *par excellence* (Foucault 1976), emphasizing woman's unique sexual character. Medical scientists now started to identify the "essential features that belong to her, that serve to distinguish her, that make her what she is" (T. Laqueur 1990: 5). The medical literature of this period shows a radical naturalization of femininity in which scientists reduced woman to one specific organ. In the eighteenth and nineteenth centuries scientists set out to localize the "essence" of femininity in different places in the body. Until the mid-nineteenth century, scientists considered the uterus as the seat of femininity. This conceptualization is reflected in the statement of the German poet and naturalist Johann Wolfgang von Goethe (1749–1832): Der Hauptpunkt der ganzen weiblichen Existenz ist die Gebaermutter (The main point (or the essence) of the entire female existence is the womb) (Medvei 1983: 213).

In the middle of the nineteenth century, medical attention began to shift from the uterus to the ovaries, which came to be regarded as largely autonomous control centers of reproduction in the female animal, while in humans they were thought to be the "essence" of femininity itself (Gallagher and Laqueur 1987: 27). In 1848, Virchow (1817–1885), often portrayed as the founding father of physiology, characterized the function of the ovaries:

> It has been completely wrong to regard the uterus as the characteristic organ.... The womb, as part of the sexual canal, of the whole apparatus of reproduction, is merely an organ of secondary importance. Remove the ovary, and we shall have before us a masculine woman, an ugly half-form with the coarse and harsh form, the heavy bone formation, the moustache, the rough voice, the flat chest, the sour and egoistic mentality and the distorted outlook ... in short, all that we admire and respect in woman as womanly, is merely dependent on her ovaries.
>
> (Medvei 1983: 215)

The search for the female organ *par excellence* was not just a theoretical endeavor. The place in the body where the "essence" of femininity was located became the object of surgical interventions. The ovaries, perceived as the "organs of crises", became the paradigmatic object of the medical specialty of gynecology that was established in the late nineteenth century (Honegger 1991: 209, 211). The medical attention given to the ovaries resulted in the widespread practice of surgical operations for removal of the ovaries in many European countries, as well as in the United States. In the 1870s and 1880s, thousands of women were subjected to this drastic procedure for the treatment of menstrual irregularities and various neuroses (Corner 1965: 4).

Early in the twentieth century, the "essence" of femininity came to be located not in an organ but in chemical substances: sex hormones. The new field of sex endocrinology introduced the concept of "female" and "male" sex hormones as chemical messengers of femininity and masculinity. This hormonally constructed concept of the body has developed into one of the dominant modes of thinking about the biological roots of sex differences. Many types of behavior, roles, functions and characteristics considered as typically male or female in western culture have been ascribed to hormones.[12] In this process, the female body, but not the male

feminist shortcomings

meanings and theories. The feminist project in science depicts science only in terms of texts and ideas, thus neglecting the material aspects of science;[19] while precisely these material aspects are major characteristics of the biomedical sciences. Science is not just words. When we enter a biomedical laboratory, we see how scientists use microscopes, test tubes, X-ray apparatus, staining techniques, etc. Once we are aware of this, it seems implausible to reduce science primarily to theoretical interests. The development of scientific knowledge depends not only on ideas, ideologies or theories, but also on complex instruments, research materials, careful preparatory procedures and testing practices.[20] Moreover, as biomedical discourses are the product of material conditions, they have fundamental material effects as well. The biomedical sciences have a material authority *biomedical authority* that is manifest in the form of diagnostic tools, screening tests, drugs and other regulatory devices. This is a social reality with which millions of people who experience sickness are confronted in their daily lives, a reality that should not be neglected in feminist studies of science. I therefore chose to focus particularly on the materiality of discourse-building, which leads us to the down-to-earth activities of scientists, such as collecting urine and ovaries, as well as the poetically unpromising testing practices at the laboratory bench and in the clinic.

The design of this book is as follows. Chapter 2 focuses on the role of cultural notions in the development of hypotheses and theories in early research on sex hormones. The following chapters focus more specifically on the material conditions for the study of sex hormones and the social networks in which the study of sex hormones took place. Chapter 3 analyzes the experimental practices of hormonal research, which contributed to changing the meanings and practices that became associated with the female and the male body. Chapters 4, 5 and 6 extend the analysis to groups outside the laboratory. Chapter 4 analyzes the role of research materials in structuring the relationships between the laboratory, the clinic and the pharmaceutical company, and describes how the study of female sex hormones – and not male sex hormones – gradually developed into big science and big business. Chapter 5 describes how sex hormones were made into specialized drugs, and analyzes how it happened that the female body became increasingly subjected to hormonal treatment. Chapters 4 and 5 focus more exclusively on the Dutch situation. Dutch laboratory scientists, as well as Dutch pharmaceutical entrepreneurs, were major actors in the emerging field of sex endocrinology. The Pharmaco-Therapeutic Laboratory at the University of Amsterdam, headed by the physician and pharmacologist Ernst Laqueur, was one of the leading research groups in the 1920s and 1930s. This research group was among the first to isolate pure crystalline estrogenic hormone, and the first to isolate the "male" sex hormone testosterone (Parkes 1966). Organon, the Dutch pharmaceutical company founded in 1923, was the major producer of estrogens throughout the world until the Second World

War (Tausk 1978: 35) and still is among the top three in the present world market for hormonal contraceptives (Anonymous 1992). Chapter 6 takes up the course of history of sex endocrinology in the late 1950s, when American scientists transformed sex hormones into the contraceptive pill. It describes the infrastructural arrangements in which women of color became the guinea-pigs of one of the most revolutionary drugs in the history of medicine.[21] Chapter 7, finally, evaluates the major conclusions that can be drawn from this story of sex hormones for the continuing debate about science, sex and the body.

2 The birth of sex hormones

Nowadays, we can hardly imagine a world without hormones. We have to travel in time to find other worlds that are not yet inhabited by them. Imagine a scene on a lazy Sunday afternoon in the late nineteenth century. Ladies are chattering about the exciting events of the past days. If we could eavesdrop on these conversations, we would hear detailed, intimate accounts of how these women try to cope with daily life. Maybe we are lucky and we can overhear them exchanging experiences about pregnancy and delivery. We will never know precisely which words women used in those days to express themselves, but we know one thing for sure: women did not refer to hormones to explain their lives. Simply because the very word hormones did not exist in the nineteenth century.

Where does the concept of hormones, particularly sex hormones, come from? How did it become included in the medical discourses about the body? What inspired scientists to develop a totally new model for understanding bodies? Obviously, scientists who introduce new concepts into science do not start from scratch. Or to paraphrase Nelson Goodman: "scientific development always starts from worlds already on hand" (Goodman 1978: 6). I would like to know which worlds inspired scientists to introduce the concept of sex hormones. As I indicated in the Introduction, Fleck's concept of prescientific ideas is useful here (Fleck 1979: 23–27). It made me wonder whether the introduction of the concept of sex hormones was linked to any previously existing beliefs about women and men; and if so, how did these prescientific ideas then become integrated into the emerging field of sex endocrinology? Using Fleck's notion of prescientific ideas, I shall trace which cultural ideas became embodied in the concept of sex hormones and how and to what extent scientists actively transformed these ideas, once they were incorporated in research practice. My strategy is to focus on the different disciplines that became involved in hormone research. Sex endocrinology, like other fields in the life sciences at the turn of the twentieth century, was characterized by two different approaches: a biological approach and a chemical approach (Clarke 1985: 390; Kohler 1982). In the early years, the study of sex hormones was dominated by scientists who adopted a biological style:

physiologists, gynecologists, anatomists and zoologists.[1] In the 1920s, chemical approaches came to dominate the field.[2] I shall examine the extent to which differences in disciplinary styles may account for the transformation of prescientific ideas.

Finally, I shall evaluate the impact of the introduction of the concept of sex hormones on the conceptualization of sex differences. What were the consequences of this new approach in the study of the human body? I describe how sex endocrinology caused a revolutionary change in the study of sex differences and led to a conceptualization of sex that meant a definitive break with prescientific ideas about the female and the male body.

HOW THE CONCEPT OF SEX HORMONES ORIGINATED

The first use of the term "hormone" can be traced back to Britain. In 1905, Ernest H. Starling, professor in physiology at University College in London, introduced the concept of hormones:

> These chemical messengers ... or "hormones" as we may call them, have to be carried from the organ where they are produced to the organ which they affect, by means of the blood stream, and the continually recurring physiological needs of the organism must determine their production and circulation through the body.
>
> (Starling 1905)

The concept of hormones as potent substances regulating physical processes in organisms implied a drastic change in the paradigm of physiology. Edward Schaefer, professor at University College in London, evaluated this shift as follows:

> The Old Physiology was based, as we have seen, on nervous regulation; the New Physiology is based on chemical regulation.... The changes of physiology which have resulted from this knowledge constitute not merely an advance in degree but an alteration in character.... We must in future explain physiological changes in terms of chemical regulation as well as nervous regulation.
>
> (Edward Schaefer as cited in Medvei 1983: 339)

The "New Physiology" enabled scientists to conceptualize the development of organisms in terms of chemical agencies, rather than just nervous stimuli. The chemical messengers believed to originate from the gonads (sex glands) were designated sex hormones, with male sex hormone designating the secretion of the testis and female sex hormone designating ovarian secretion. With the introduction of the concept of sex hormones scientists suggested that they had found the key to understanding what made a man a man and a woman a woman. In the General Biological Introduction to the first textbook of sex endocrinology, *Sex and Internal*

Secretions, the French-Canadian zoologist Frank R. Lillie evaluated this rapidly expanding research field:

> One of the most interesting and promising lines of experimental bio-logical investigations of the present century has been in the biology of sex. It has been discovered that sex characteristics in general are subject to certain simple mechanisms of control that operate through-out the life history, and which determine whether male or female characters shall develop in the individual. ... The mechanisms of con-trol are exceedingly simple compared with the sex machinery itself. ... This book deals predominantly with a method of control of sex charac-ters which is especially characteristic of vertebrates including man, mediated by hormones circulating in the blood. Of these, the specific internal secretions of the testis, or male sex hormone, and the spe-cific internal secretion of the cortex of the ovary, or female sex hor-mone, are the most important, and probably occur in all vertebrates.
>
> (Lillie 1939: 5-6)

In the same textbook Lillie described the function of sex hormones:

> As there are two sets of sex characters, so there are two sex hor-mones, the male hormone controlling the "dependent" male characters, and the female determining the "dependent" female characters.
>
> (Lillie 1939: 11)

Sex hormones were thus conceptualized as the chemical messengers of masculinity and femininity.

To what extent were these developments linked to any prescientific ideas? The idea of testes and ovaries as agents of masculinity and feminin-ity can be traced back to several periods in which these ideas emerged, prior to the hormonal era.

The idea that the ovaries are in one way or another related to female sexual development can be traced back as far as Aristotle. In his *History of Animals* Aristotle wrote that "the ovaries of sows are excised with the view of quenching in them sexual appetites and of stimulating growth in size and fatness" (Aristotle as cited in Corner 1965: 3). Aristotle was referring here to the custom of removing ovaries in domestic animals, a widespread practice among European farmers in the Middle Ages, that seems to have been kept in use till the late nineteenth century. The idea that the ovaries are somehow linked to female sexuality remained, how-ever, for a long time restricted to the domain of agricultural practices (Corner 1965: 4).

Let us first focus our attention on the prescientific precursors of the concept of male sex hormones, before tracing how the idea of ovaries as agents of femininity became incorporated in the life sciences. The idea that the male gonads are the seat of masculinity is a very old one. From the earliest times, the testis has been linked with male sexuality, longevity and bravery. Greeks and Romans used preparations made from goat or wolf testes as sexual stimulants. The seventeenth century brought a revival of these ancient ideas of virility. In this period, the prescientific idea of testes as agents of masculinity became for the first time incorporated into medical science. European reformers, like the physician Paracelsus, used testes extracts in the treatment of "imbecility of the instruments of generation." The official pharmacopoeia of the London College of Physicians of 1676 gave directions for the extraction of animal reproductive organs as a treatment for numerous illnesses and as sexual stimulants. In the eighteenth century, belief in the testis as the controller of virility was abandoned to the realm of folk-wisdom and quackery. By 1800, testicular extracts had disappeared from the official pharmacopoeias in Europe. The belief in the testis as agent of masculinity remained, however, very much alive in popular culture. Although the medical profession strongly disapproved of testicular therapy, potions made from testis extracts were among the wares of eighteenth-century quacks and were quite popular all over Europe.[3]

How did the pre-ideas of testes and ovaries as seats of masculinity and femininity become integrated into the modern life sciences? The most conspicuous actor in advocating the doctrine of the gonads was the French physiologist Charles-Edouard Brown-Séquard. In 1889, Brown-Séquard addressed his colleagues at the Société de Biologie in Paris, reporting the results of self-medication in which he had treated himself with injections prepared by crushing guinea-pigs' and dogs' testicles, resulting in "a marked renewal of vigour and mental clarity." He also reported the practices of a midwife in Paris, who treated women with the filtered juice of guinea-pigs' ovaries for "hysteria, various uterine affections, and debility due to age" (Corner 1965: 5). On this occasion Brown-Séquard suggested that the testes produced a secretion that controlled the development of the male organism. These "internal secretions" might be discovered by using extracts in treatment for certain diseases.[4] Brown-Séquard's advocacy gave rise to a renewed interest in the 1890s in what was now called "organotherapy": the use of extracts of animal organs as therapeutic agents.[5]

The scientific community reacted for the most part with hostility to Brown-Séquard's claims. In their eyes the clock was being put back to the dark ages of quackery. On the other hand, Brown-Séquard, as the successor to Claude Bernard at the Collège de France, was considered a distinguished neurophysiologist (Hamilton 1986: 12,15). Moreover, Brown-Séquard's ideas harmonized with Victorian notions of masculinity. He suggested that the secretions of the testis were present in the seminal fluid containing sperm. In this manner, Brown-Séquard linked his ideas to the then popular notion that loss of semen, through sexual intercourse or, even worse, masturbation, was weakening the male. Brown-Séquard's claims thus not only reflected prescientific ideas about the power of the testis that can be traced back to early civilization, but also reflected the sexual assumptions of Victorian days (Hamilton 1986: 16).

If we want to trace how the prescientific idea of the ovaries as the seat of femininity became integrated into the center of the life sciences, we have to direct our attention to another place: the gynecological clinic. It was through changes in medical practice that the prescientific idea of ovaries as agents of femininity became incorporated into scientific theory and practice. Until the mid-nineteenth century, medical scientists studying the female body focussed their attention primarily on the womb. The uterus was known several millennia before the ovary (the "female testicle") was described as an anatomic unit.[6] Scientists located the essence of femininity in the uterus. Beginning in the middle of the nineteenth century, medical attention gradually shifted from the uterus to the ovaries. The ovaries came to be regarded as the essence of femininity itself: the study of these organs would lead to an understanding of woman's whole being, including all women's diseases. (Gallagher and Laqueur 1987: 27). In gynecological textbooks the ovary was described as "the organ of crisis which is missing in the male body." This shift from the uterus to the ovaries provided the gynecological profession with their own "paradigm-specific" organ which enabled them to delineate the boundaries between gynecology and obstetrics, the profession that focused primarily on the uterus (Honegger 1991: 82–83).

In this period the role of the ovaries was yet described in terms of chemical substances, but rather in the then popular terms of regulation by the nervous system. Gynecologists were the first to introduce the idea that ovaries secreted chemical substances that regulate the development of the female body (Medvei 1983: 215). They were already familiar with the changes in the body that followed the removal of ovaries, due to the widespread medical practice of surgical operations for the removal of the ovaries in the late nineteenth century (Corner 1965: 4; T. Laqueur 1990: 176). Two Viennese gynecologists, Emil Knauer and Josef Halban, described the secretion of chemical substances by the ovaries as early as 1896 and 1900. Gynecologists were thus the first to recognize the relevance of Brown-Séquard's theory of "internal secretions" to the female sex glands.[7] This branch of the medical profession came under the spell of the glands because of their therapeutic promises. Gynecologists were particularly attracted to the concept of female sex hormones because it promised a better understanding and therefore greater medical control over the complex of disorders in their female patients frequently associated with the ovaries, such as disturbances in menstruation and various diseases described as "nervous" in medical literature. Moreover, by linking female disorders to female sex hormones, "women's problems" remained inside the domain of the gynecologists.

THE EMERGENCE OF SEX ENDOCRINOLOGY

In the first decade of the twentieth century, the study of sex hormones developed into a major field of research that became known as sex endocrinology.[8] The concept of sex hormones as agents of masculinity and femininity functioned as a paradigm, focusing previously scattered research around a generally accepted theory. Compared with gynecologists, physiologists were relatively slow to recognize the relevance of the theory of internal secretions for the sex glands. One of the main reasons for this was the association of the sex glands with human sexuality and reproduction, an area that previously had been taboo in biomedical research. This negative association was reinforced by the therapeutic claims of Brown-Séquard about the effects of testis extracts on the sexual activity of men, claims that caused a controversy among clinicians and laboratory scientists. Physiologists who took up the study of ovary and testes preparations did so cautiously, avoiding association with these therapeutic claims. Obviously, the subject was more legitimate for gynecologists (Borell 1985: 2).[9]

After the turn of the twentieth century, physiologists also gradually came under the spell of the gonads. Schaefer's laboratory in London was one of the first physiological laboratories that took up the study of the ovaries (Borell 1985: 13). The physiologists were particularly interested in the study of the glands because the concept of hormones provided a new model for understanding the physiology of the body. In the first decade of the twentieth century, physiologists included the study of the ovaries and testes as a branch of general biology (Corner 1965: 7). Hereby the traditional borders between two different groups of actors – the physiologists and the gynecologists – changed drastically. Before the turn of the twentieth century the study of ovaries, particularly in relation to female disorders, had been the exclusive field of gynecologists. With the introduction of the concept of sex hormones, laboratory scientists explicitly linked female disorders with laboratory practice, thus entering a domain that had traditionally been the reserve of gynecologists. Whereas gynecologists were particularly interested in the functions of the ovaries in order to control all kinds of disorders ascribed to ovarian malfunction, physiologists had a broader interest in the role of the ovaries and testes in the development of the body.

The concept of hormones triggered a new experimental approach in laboratory science. At the turn of the twentieth century scientists began to search actively for the chemical substances in the sex glands using the techniques of castration and transplantation. In this surgical approach, scientists removed ovaries and testes from animals like rabbits and guinea-pigs, cut them into fragments, and reimplanted them into the same individuals at locations other than their normal positions in the body. With these experiments scientists tested the concept of hormones as agents having control over physical processes without the mediation of nervous tissue. In transplantation the nervous tissue of the glands was dissected, so the effects of the reimplanted glands on the development of the organism had to take place through another medium, such as the blood (Borell 1985).

The acceptance of the hormonal theory in the biological sciences was facilitated by the fact that it fitted into a major debate among biologists about the sexual development of organisms. In the 1910s, the topic of sexual development was most controversial, particularly between physiologists and geneticists. Physiologists at that time suggested that the determination of sexual characteristics is affected by environmental and physiological conditions during the development of the embryo. Geneticists suggested however that sex is irrevocably fixed at conception by nuclear elements: the sex chromosomes.[10]

With the introduction of the concept of sex hormones, sex endocrinologists claimed they had found the missing link between the genetic and the physiological models of sex determination. In 1916, Frank Lillie provided arguments for the role of sex hormones as well as sex chromosomes in the sexual development of higher animals by studying intersexes in cows. Lillie looked at the anatomical characteristics of the freemartin, the sexually abnormal co-twin of a male calf, usually possessing female as well as male external genitalia. Lillie suggested that the freemartin, a "natural experiment," is genetically female but that "a powerful blood-born chemical produced in the male had altered the sex that the genes intended for the freemartin". Lillie thus suggested that "the intentions of the genes must always be carried through by appropriate hormones developed in the gonad."[11]

This suggestion provided geneticists and sex endocrinologists with arguments to demarcate the fields of the two young sciences with respect to the study of sex, a demarcation coined with the concepts of sex determination and sexual differentiation. Geneticists focussed on the study of sex determination, defined in *Sex and Internal Secretions* as "the establishment of internal conditions leading to the development of one or the other set of sex characters". Sex endocrinologists restricted their research to the study of sexual differentiation: "the development of sexual characteristics in the course of the individual's life history." Lillie described this demarcation of the domains of genetics and sex endocrinology as follows:

> It is clear that we must make a radical distinction between sex determination and sex differentiation. In most cases the factors of sex determination are chromosomal, and subject to the usual laws of Mendelian inheritance. . . . In the higher vertebrates, the mechanism of sex differentiation is taken over by extracellular agents, the male and the female sex hormones.

> (Lillie 1939: 7–8)[12]

In the early decades of the twentieth century sexual development came thus to be defined as the result of two processes: sex determination regulated by genetic factors, and sexual differentiation influenced by hormonal factors.

In the 1920s, biochemists became involved in the study of sex hormones. Following advances in organic chemistry in the late 1910s, the surgical approach of transplanting gonads was replaced by chemical extraction of the gonads. The introduction of the chemical approach into the study of sex hormones was – compared with other fields – somewhat belated. This delay was partly due to technical problems. In the 1910s, biochemists were preoccupied with proteins. In this period the biochemists had "neither the incentive nor the information" to enter the field of sex hormone research. This situation changed in the 1920s when lipid chemistry emerged as a new line of inquiry in biochemistry. In the 1920s, sex hormones were classified as steroids, a class of substances that could be extracted with the same solvents applied in extracting lipids, thus providing biochemists with both the information and the tools to enter the study of sex hormones (Long Hall 1975: 83).

In addition to clinicians and laboratory scientists, the emerging field of sex endocrinology also attracted a third group to the scene: the pharmaceutical industry. The manufacturing of extracts from animal organs offered a new and promising line of production. Pharmaceutical companies started producing ovary and testes preparations, and not without success. At the turn of the century the advertising pages of medical journals were full of recommendations for the prescription of these preparations under a wide variety of trade names, indicating a flourishing trade in "biologicals" (Corner 1965: 6). Many researchers involved in the study of sex hormones worked in close cooperation with pharmaceutical companies. This issue will be dealt with in further detail in Chapter 4.

SEX HORMONES AS DUALISTIC AGENTS OF SEX

By 1910, the prescientific idea of the gonads as agents of sex differences had been transformed into the concept of sex hormones as chemical messengers of masculinity and femininity. With this conceptualization, sex endocrinologists reformulated the cultural notion of gonads as the seat of masculinity and femininity. Sex endocrinologists focussed their attention on the secretions of the gonads, rather than on the gonads themselves. In other respects, the scientific conceptualization of sex remained very close to common-sense opinions about masculinity and femininity. In the early period of sex endocrinology, the concept of sex hormones was straightforward and simple: there existed just two sex hormones, one per sex. In the period between 1905 and 1920, scientists defined sex hormones as exclusively sex specific in origin and function. With this conceptualization sex endocrinologists suggested that sex had to be considered as a strictly dualistic concept.

This conceptualization not only harmonized with the prescientific idea of a sexual duality located in the gonads, but also found a ready acceptance given the cultural notions of masculinity and femininity of the day. In this period the dominant cultural idea of sex was determined by the Doctrine of the Two Sexes, a concept of sex developed in Victorian times but still prevalent in the opening decades of the twentieth century. According to this doctrine, women's activities were in most respects the opposite of those of men. Therefore female and male were understood as opposite categories, not as two independent or complementary dimensions (Lewin 1984: 169–170).

The idea of female and male as opposite categories was further reinforced by those sex endocrinologists who advocated the idea of sex antagonism. Some scientists – anticipating the women's liberation movement at the turn of the century – had advocated the idea of sex antagonism. Among them was the British physiologist Walter Heape, who was the first to study the menstrual cycle of women in relation to the estrus cycle in animals. In 1913, Heape published a book entitled *Sex Antagonism*, an anthropological study claiming that women's biological destiny was the opposite of men's (Heape 1913). Heape refuted the claims of feminists to equal rights for women and argued that biology restricted women's destiny to motherhood. Although it was criticized for its unfounded biological determinism, Heape's colleagues subscribed to his view of the relations between the sexes. In his review of *Sex Antagonism* the British evolutionary biologist J. Arthur Thomson emphasized that it was good biology to emphasize that woman's usefulness depends on her dissimilarity to man (Thomson 1914: 346 as quoted in Long Hall 1975: 85).

In the 1910s, the Viennese gynecologist Eugen Steinach attributed the idea of sex antagonism to the concept of sex hormones. With Heape and scientists like the Dutch sexologist Van de Velde, Steinach shared a conservative reaffirmation of the traditional distinction between the sexes, emphasizing that the appropriate social roles for women were rooted in biology and opposite to men's roles (Long Hall 1976). Steinach conceptualized the organism as a system of competing forces and persuaded his colleagues that male and female gonads secreted opposite, antagonistic hormones (Long Hall 1975: 88).

In itself, the idea of sex antagonism was new to the field of sex hormones. Earlier workers like Brown-Séquard had restricted the function of sex hormones to stimulating the development of "homologous" sexual characteristics, suggesting that female sex hormones controlled female characteristics and male sex hormones male sexual characteristics. Steinach, however, attributed a double potentiality to sex hormones by suggesting that "sex hormones simultaneously stimulated homologous sexual characteristics and depressed heterologous sexual characteristics." Besides stimulating the development of female sexual characteristics, female sex hormones were thought to suppress the development of male sexual characteristics.[13]

In more popular writings on sex hormones, this supposed antagonism between both type of hormones was compared with the relationship between men and women: "the chemical war between the male and the female hormones is, as it were, a chemical miniature of the well-known eternal war between men and women" (Kruif undated: 167). The conceptualization of sex hormones as antagonists thus fitted seamlessly with Victorian notions of the proper relationship between the sexes, and was consistent with the dualistic idea that each sex had its own specific sex hormone.

The emerging field of sex endocrinology shows a striking unanimity in interpretations of the concept of sex hormones. The groups involved in research on sex hormones, during this period mainly gynecologists and some biologists (physiologists, anatomists and zoologists), basically agreed about the conceptualization of sex hormones. This unanimity changed drastically when the field became more specialized and new groups entered the arena of hormonal research. In the 1920s, there emerged a lively dispute in the scientific community about the dualistic assumption that sex hormones are strictly sex-specific in origin and function. A growing number of publications appeared contradicting the prescientific idea of a sexual duality located in the gonads and underlying the original concept of the sexual specifity of sex hormones. The next sections describe how the different disciplines involved in the study of sex hormones gradually transformed the prescientific idea of sexual duality into a new meaning of sex.

SEX-SPECIFIC ORIGIN

The first challenges to the prescientific idea of a sexual duality located in the gonads appeared in the early 1920s. In 1921, the Viennese gynecologist Otfried Fellner published an article in *Pflueger's Archiv* describing experiments with rabbits in which extracts of the testis produced effects on the growth of the uterus similar to those produced by ovarian extracts. Fellner suggested that the testis of the rabbit obviously contained female sex hormones (Fellner 1921: 189).[14] It took several years before this report evoked reactions from his colleagues. Remarkably, this response came from the "newcomers" in the field of sex endocrinology: the biochemists. The biochemical focus on the chemical identification and isolation of sex hormones generated a new set of needs for raw materials, amongst others urine (Clarke 1987b: 331).[15] In this biochemical search for new resources to obtain female sex hormone (to replace the expensive ovaries), scientists reported the presence of female sex hormones in men. Ernst Laqueur's research group at the Pharmaco-Therapeutic Laboratory of the University of Amsterdam – the Amsterdam School, as they were known by other scientists – reported in 1927 that female sex hormone was present not only in the testis but also in the urine of "normal, healthy" men. (E. Laqueur *et al.* 1927b: 1,859).

What really made an impact was an article which appeared in 1934 in *Nature* by the German gynecologist Bernhard Zondek, then working at the Biochemical Institute of the University of Stockholm (Figure 2.1).[16]

FEBRUARY 10, 1934   **N A T U R E**

Letters to the Editor

[The Editor does not hold himself responsible for opinions expressed by his correspondents. Neither can he undertake to return, nor to correspond with the writers of, rejected manuscripts intended for this or any other part of NATURE. *No notice is taken of anonymous communications.]*

Mass Excretion of Œstrogenic Hormone in the Urine of the Stallion

IN earlier investigations[1] it was shown that the largest quantities of œstrogenic hormone (folliculin— s. œstrin) are excreted in the urine of pregnant mares (100,000 mouse units per litre). I found this also to be the case in other equines (ass, zebra) during pregnancy, whereas, in the non-pregnant state, the excretion of hormone both in equines and in other mammals is very small, at most 0·5 per cent in comparison with that of the gravid animal. <u>Curiously enough</u>, as a result of further investigations, it appears that in the urine of the stallion also, very large quantities of œstrogenic hormone are eliminated.

Figure 2.1 Bernhard Zondek's Letter to the Editor of *Nature* in which he announces the presence of "œstrogenic hormone" in the urine of the stallion. *Source*: Zondek (1934a)

In this article, entitled "Mass excretion of œstrogenic hormones in urine of the stallion", Zondek described his observations as follows:

> Curiously enough, as a result of further investigations, it appears that in the urine of the stallion also, very large quantities of œstrogenic hormone are eliminated. . . . I found this mass excretion of hormone only in the male and not in the female horse. The determination of

the hormone content, therefore, makes hormonic recognition of sex possible in the urine of a horse. In this connexion we find the paradox that the male sex is recognized by a high œstrogenic hormone content.

(Zondek 1934a)

In the same publication Zondek reported that "the testis of the horse is the richest tissue known to contain œstrogenic hormone." One month later he published a second article in *Nature* describing the identity and the origin of female sex hormones in males.[17] Zondek's observations were startling at the time. Who could have expected that the gonads of a male animal would turn out to be the richest source of female sex hormone ever observed?

The female of the species did not escape this confusion: in the same period, reports were published of the presence of male sex hormones in female organisms – but it is interesting that this phenomenon received far less attention. The articles indexed in the *Quarterly Cumulative Index Medicus* show that the number of articles written on females is considerably less than on males.[18] The first publication reporting the presence of male sex hormone in female organisms was published in 1931 by the German gynecologist Siebke. In 1932, this observation was confirmed by Elisabeth Dingemanse, a biochemist from the Amsterdam School (Jongh 1934b). In the years to follow, the British physiologist Hill published a series of contributions under the flagrant title, *Ovaries secrete male hormone* (Evans 1939: 597).

The above observations contradicted the original concept of the sexual specificity of sex hormones. What label should be attached to substances isolated from male organisms possessing properties classified as being specific to female sex hormones, and vice versa? Scientists decided to name these substances female sex hormones and male sex hormones, thus abandoning the criteria of exclusively sex-specific origin. Female sex hormones were no longer conceptualized as restricted to female organisms, and male sex hormones were no longer thought to be present only in males. Here we see how scientists gradually moved away from the prescientific idea that the essence of femininity is located in the ovaries, while the testes are the seat of masculinity. This shift in conceptualization led to a drastic break with the dualistic cultural notion of masculinity and femininity that had existed for centuries.

Because the prescientific idea of a sexual duality located in the gonads had dominated research for years, scientists were rather taken aback by the idea that female sex hormone could also be found in male bodies.[19] In the first reports these results were evaluated as "one of the most surprising observations in the sex hormone field" and "a strange and apparently anomalous discovery"; the reports contained phrases like "curiously enough," "unexpected observation" and "paradoxical finding" (Frank 1929: 292; Jongh 1934b: 1,209; Parkes 1938; Zondek 1934a: 209).

Many scientists found their own results so surprising that they felt obliged to emphasize the fact that they had used the urine and blood of "normal, healthy men and women." In *The Female Sex Hormone*, Robert Frank, a gynecologist at Mount Sinai Hospital in New York, legitimized the identity of his test subjects by the statement that he had observed female sex hormones in the bodies of males 'whose masculine character and ability to impregnate females" were unquestioned (Frank 1929: 120). Other scientists, however, concluded that the tested subjects, though apparently normal, were "latent hermaphrodites" (Parkes 1966: 26).

SOURCE AND IDENTITY OF "HETEROSEXUAL HORMONES"

Confronted with these unexpected data, scientists started looking for a plausible theory to explain the source and identity of these "heterosexual hormones" (as female sex hormones in male organisms, and vice versa, were named) (Jongh 1934b: 1,209). In the 1930s, different hypotheses were proposed to explain the presence of female sex hormones in male organisms. In some of these hypotheses, scientists tried hard to maintain the dualistic conceptualization of sex according to which male and female were defined as mutually exclusive categories.

In 1929, Robert Frank suggested that female sex hormones were not produced by the male body itself, but that they originated from food (Frank 1929: 293). In the late 1930s, this hypothesis was criticized as implausible by, among others, the Amsterdam School (Dingemanse *et al.* 1937). Despite this criticism, the food hypothesis remained popular. In *Sex and Internal Secretions*, the food hypothesis is advanced without paying attention to the critical notes of the author of the cited paper:

> Following the demonstration of the wide occurrence of estrogens in foods, it became apparent that estrogens in male urine need not necessarily imply their secretion in the male body. Eng (1934) reported that when a young man was placed on an estrogen-free diet, the excretion of estrogen in both urine and faeces dropped to 3 mouse units per day. On a standard diet, between 13 and 44 units per day could be recovered from the urine of the same man.
>
> (Allen *et al.* 1939: 561)

The food hypothesis seems to have been postulated only for the presence of female sex hormone in male organisms: no reports were published attempting to explain the presence of male sex hormones in females by the intake of male hormones from food.

In contrast with Frank, British scientists like the biologists Nancy and Robert Callow and Alan Parkes from the National Institute for Medical Research in Hampstead, London, suggested that male bodies should be considered capable of producing female sex hormones and proposed the adrenals as one of the sites of the production of sex hormones. (Callow and Callow 1938; Parkes 1937). The adrenal hypothesis was still consistent with the prescientific idea of a sexual duality, in which it was impossible to consider the gonads capable of excretion of both sex hormones. In 1951, Samuel de Jongh, one of the laboratory scientists of the Amsterdam School, evaluated the proposal of the adrenal hypothesis as follows:

> By proposing the hypothesis of an extra-gonadal source to explain the presence of female sex hormones in male bodies, scientists could avoid the necessity to attribute the secretion of male sex hormones to the ovary.
>
> (Jongh 1951: 20)

It was the gonadal hypothesis, suggested by Zondek in 1934, that first broke with the dualistic concept of sex hormones. In this hypothesis it was proposed that the regular occurrence of female sex hormones in male organisms was the result of the conversion from male sex hormones into female ones (Zondek 1934b). The idea of conversion was strongly advocated by biochemists, who posited a close interrelationship between male and female sex hormones and brought about the general acceptance of the idea that the gonads produce both type of sex hormones. After 1937, the adrenals and the gonads of both sexes were considered as the sites of production of male as well as female sex hormones (Kochakian 1938; Parkes 1938).

This succession of hypotheses illustrates how the prescientific idea of a sexual duality located in the gonads was gradually reshaped into a new conceptualization of sex differences. In this period, scientists definitely broke with the cultural notion that the essence of femininity and masculinity was located only in the gonads. They suggested that the chemical messengers of masculinity and femininity were present in the adrenals as well as in the gonads of all organisms, rather than being restricted to the gonads of one sex. In the 1930s, scientists reshaped the original dualistic assumption of the sex-specific origin of sex hormones into a conceptualization in which the categories male and female were no longer considered mutually exclusive. By the end of the 1930s, scientists supported the idea that male bodies could possess female sex hormones and vice versa, thus for the first time combining the categories of male and female into one sex.

The debate over the sex-specific origin of sex hormones shows how the different disciplines played different roles in this controversy. Although the presence of female sex hormones in male bodies was reported by gynecologists and biologists, the biochemists took a key position in the debate on the sex-specific origin of sex hormones, as the following citation from the Amsterdam School illustrates:

> In the second place I want to reflect on the question of whether the estrus-producing substance that is present in the organs and body fluids

of men, and apparently has a function there, is really female sex hormone. In fact we know nothing more than that it can cause the same effects as female sex hormone. An identification can only be possible after the chemical isolation of this oestrus-producing substance from male products, which has not yet been done.

(Jongh 1934b: 1,213)

Prior to the 1930s, the question of the identity of sex hormones could be addressed only by using the techniques of biological assays. Substances isolated from male urine which passed the biological assays specific for female sex hormones were defined as female sex hormones. It was only after 1929 that scientists could assess the identity of sex hormones with chemical methods, thanks to developments in organic chemistry in the area of steroid and lipoid compounds. Sex hormones – classified as steroids – could now be chemically identified and isolated (Long Hall 1975). Female sex hormones were first chemically isolated from the urine of horses and pregnant women in 1929. In 1932, English and German chemists classified female sex hormones as steroid substances, and a colorimetric test was developed to detect the presence of female sex hormone in organisms (Walsh 1985). Male sex hormones were first isolated from men's urine in 1931 and were classified two years later in the same group of chemical substances as female sex hormones: the steroids.

In 1938, the Amsterdam School finally reported the isolation of female sex hormone from male urine. The delay had been mainly caused by the limited availability of raw material, a general obstacle to the chemical isolation of sex hormones, which could be surmounted only by scientists working in close cooperation with pharmaceutical companies. Elisabeth Dingemanse explained the problem in an article in *Nature* as follows:

The necessity arose shortly afterwards of identifying these active substances chemically. The small amounts in which these active substances occur in adult male urine has so far made this impossible. . . . Through the intervention of the N.V. Organon-Oss, for which we take this opportunity of expressing our thanks, it has been possible for us to process 17,000 litres of male urine. . . . In this way we succeeded in obtaining 6 milligrams of a single crystalline substance. This proved to be identical with oestrone (female sex hormone).

(Dingemanse *et al.* 1928: 927)

Thus, the biochemists claimed to possess a definitive answer to the question of the identity of female sex hormone in male organisms. They defined female and male sex hormones as closely related chemical compounds, differing in just one hydroxyl group, which could be detected by chemical methods in both sexes. In this manner they broke with the dualistic concept of male and female as mutually exclusive categories (Figure 2.2).

Index to elucidate the chemical relationships between sex hormones

I. Oestrogene groep.

oestron

oestradiol

oestriol

II. Kamgroei groep.

androsteron

androstandiol

androstendion

testosteron

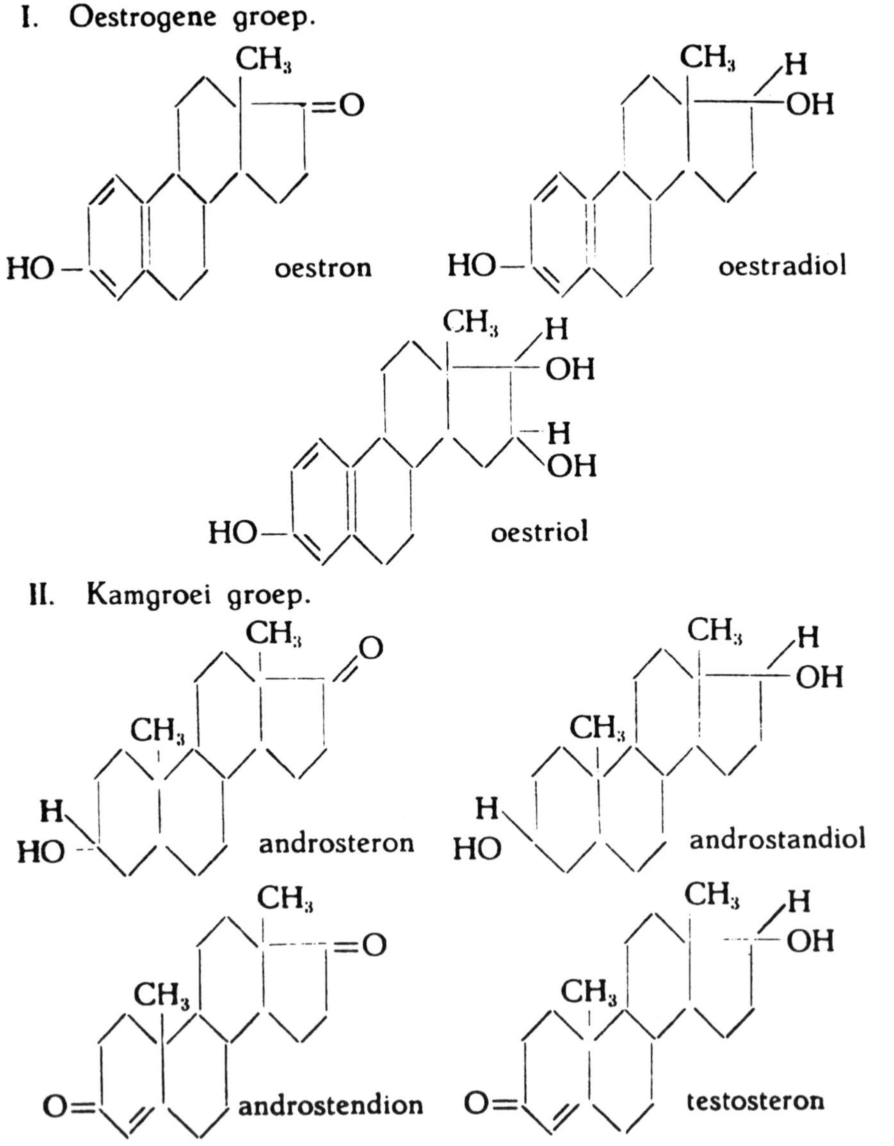

Figure 2.2 Structural formulae of the "œstrogenic hormones" and the "comb-growth hormones" to show the chemical relationships between sex hormones.
Source: J. Freud (1936)

THE FUNCTION OF HORMONES

The dispute over the sexual specificity of sex hormones did not only address the origin of sex hormones. In the 1920s, the function of "hetero-sexual" hormones was also frequently discussed. If female sex hormones were present in males, should the concept of an exclusively sex-specific function of sex hormones then be reconsidered as well? Scientists questioned whether female sex hormones had any function in the development of male organisms and vice versa. This section analyzes the positions the different disciplines involved in the study of sex hormones took in the debate about the sex-specific function of sex hormones.

The debate about the sex-specific function of sex hormones developed along lines similar to the discussion about the origin of sex hormones. Initially, scientists adhered to the prescientific notion of sexual duality. This assumption made it difficult to conceive of any function for hetero-sexual hormones at all, and therefore different hypotheses were proposed suggesting a functionless presence of the hormones. In 1929, the Amsterdam School suggested that female sex hormones probably had no function in the male body, because the concentration of female sex hormone in males was too small (Jongh *et al.* 1929: 772); in this period the amount of female sex hormone was thought to be considerably less in males than in females.

The assumption that female sex hormones had no function in male bodies directed research throughout the 1920s. In 1934, the Amsterdam School described how in 1928 they had observed the growth of the seminal vesicles in castrated rats after treatment with female sex hormones, but they had simply overlooked this function of female sex hormone in male animals. They described this observation as follows:

> Menformon (female sex hormone) – also the completely pure preparation – enlarges the seminal vesicles of animals castrated when they were young. Although this enlargement does not develop into the adult size of the seminal vesicles, this enlargement is beyond dispute. We had observed this enlargement already for years. However, we had neglected this observation because we thought it fell within the margin of error. Freud[20] and de Jongh made this observation in several different experiments. Also outside our laboratory [here the authors referred to the German scientist Loewe] the same observation was made, but was attributed to the presence of small amounts of male sex hormones in the ovarian extracts. From histological analysis I learned (and I had the pleasure of convincing Professor Loewe during a visit to our laboratory) that this conception is not right. Female sex hormone does enlarge the seminal vesicle, but in its own specific way. Male sex hormones stimulate the growth of epithelial parts and female sex hormones stimulate the growth of non-epithelial parts of the seminal vesicles.
>
> (Jongh 1934b: 1,209)

The concept of sexual specificity also structured the debate about the function of "heterosexual" hormones in human bodies. Clinicians suggested that female sex hormones had no function in the normal development of male bodies. Instead, they conceptualized female sex hormones as agents that caused diseases, in particular sexual and psychological disorders. Others suggested that female sex hormones affected a specifically female development, thus focusing research on homosexuality.[21] The issue of hormones and homosexuality will be elaborated further in Chapter 3.

By the end of the 1930s, scientists had largely accepted the idea that "heterosexual hormones" have a function in the normal development of male organisms, thus abandoning the dualistic concept of an exclusive sex-specific hormonal function. This led, in turn, to the reconsideration of another assumption in the original conceptualization of sex hormones. At the moment that the idea of the sex-specific function of sex hormones was overthrown, scientists questioned the concept of sex antagonism as well. If female sex hormones were present in male bodies, it was hard to maintain the idea of an antagonistic effect on the development of male sexual characteristics. In the early 1930s, the idea of an antagonism between male and female sex hormones was widely disputed. In this debate we see again how the disciplinary background of scientists structured their claims. From a chemical perspective, Ernst Laqueur, professor at the Pharmaco-Therapeutic Laboratory at the University of Amsterdam, rejected the idea of sex antagonism in 1935 as follows: "Our chemical knowledge makes the original exaggerated assumption of the antagonism between male and female substances rather unlikely" (E. Laqueur 1935).

We saw above how biochemists had defined sex hormones as chemically related compounds. In this definition it is not necessary to assume an antagonistic relationship between sex hormones; other relationships are possible as well. This enabled the Amsterdam School to emphasize a different relationship between female and male sex hormones: instead of an antagonism they reported on the cooperative actions of sex hormones in the development of male secondary sexual organs such as the seminal vesicles, the ductus deferens and the prostate gland. Other scientists reported synergistic actions of male and female sex hormones in female rats, in such processes as stimulation of the growth of the uterus, the first opening of the vagina, and changes in the uterus similar to those seen during pregnancy – processes "typical of the most female sexual function" (Korenchevsky *et al.* 1937).

In this debate about sex antagonism, we see how sex endocrinologists actively transformed the prescientific idea that femininity and masculinity reside in the gonads. The American researchers Carl Moore and Dorothy Price, both experimental biologists from the Department of Zoology of the University of Chicago, extended the conceptualization of sex from the gonads to the brain. In 1932, they postulated the idea of a feedback system between the gonads and the hypophysis – that is, they suggested that the inhibiting effects of female sex hormones on male sexual characteristics could not be understood in terms of a direct antagonistic effect on the male gonads, but rather in terms of a depressing effect of female sex hormones on the hypophysis, thus diminishing the production of male sex hormones by the gonads (Moore and Price 1932). In 1939, Frank Lillie evaluated these developments in *Sex and Internal Secretions* as follows:

> If both sex hormones were present simultaneously . . . there should be an "antagonism" of the two hormones, each striving, so to speak, to control the development of the sex character in question. Such an antagonism was in fact postulated by earlier workers in this field, e.g., Steinach, but more recent work, especially that of Moore, seems to remove the necessity of assuming any antagonism in the simultaneous action of the two hormones, by showing that each operates independently within its own field.
>
> (Lillie 1939: 12)

In the late 1930s, the hypothesis of an endocrine feedback system was gradually accepted as the theory to explain interrelations between male and female sex hormones.[22] Scientists thus transformed the prescientific idea that the essence of femininity and masculinity resides in the gonads into a conceptualization of sex that included the brain as the organ that controls sexual development. The extension of the conceptualization from the gonads to the brain also included the postulation of a new type of hormone: the gonadotropic hormones. In 1930, Bernhard Zondek, then working at the Department of Obstetrics and Gynecology at the City Hospital in Berlin, suggested that "the motor of sexual function" is located in a specific part of the hypophysis, the pituitary gland, which produces two separate chemical substances. The function scientists ascribed to these "master hormones" was to induce the gonads to produce sex hormones (Zondek 1930: 245; Zondek and Finkelstein 1966).

Additionally, scientists reshaped the prescientific idea of a sexual duality located in the gonads. Initially, scientists had translated this cultural notion into the idea that there existed just two sex hormones, one per sex. In the 1930s, scientists dropped the claim of the existence of just one single female sex hormone. Scientists now suggested that the ovaries are capable of producing two distinct types of female sex hormone. The "one hormone" doctrine was gradually replaced by the theory that different parts of the ovaries secreted two separate chemical substances. Between 1929 and 1930, three research groups in Europe and in the United States reported the isolation of chemical substances originating from the follicular fluid of the ovaries, which they named estrogenic hormones. By 1934, research groups reported the isolation of "a second female sex hormone" that, as they claimed, originated from another part of the ovaries: the corpus luteum. This hormone ecame known as progesterone. From this time onwards, the idea of a single female sex hormone finally disappeared (Parkes 1966: 21). Some scientists depicted progesterone as "the most female type" of the female sex hormones, because this hormone was considered as sexual-specific in origin (Jongh 1936: 5,370). Other scientists suggested that this "second" female sex hormone was the more masculine of the two hormones, emphasizing its similarity in function with male sex hormones (Klein and Parkes 1937).

The 1930s were tumultuous years. Scientists reconsidered earlier assumptions about the function of sex hormones as well. In the original concept, sex hormones were understood as substances that affected only those anatomical features which were related to sexual characteristics. In the 1930s, however, reports were published suggesting that the hormones were not so restricted in their function: experiments were described in which they affected the weight of the hypophysis and liver, nitrogen metabolism, and total body weight (Korenchevsky and Hall 1938: 998). As had happened before, scientists adopted a new perspective on the function of sex hormones. After 1935, sex hormones were no longer considered as exclusively sex-specific in function, nor as merely sex hormones or antagonists; instead, they were seen as substances that could generate manifold synergistic actions in both the male and the female body. In this manner, sex endocrinologists thoroughly transformed the prescientific idea of a sexual duality located in the gonads.

TERMINOLOGY AND CLASSIFICATION

In the previous sections we have seen how in the decade from 1920 to 1930 the original concept of sex hormones was transformed with regard to the basic assumptions underlying the early conceptualization of sex hormones. The question that emerges from this is whether scientists still adhered to the concept of sex hormones. Did the drastic changes in conceptualization affect in any way the very naming of sex hormones as male and female? A perusal of the publications of the 1930s suggests that the debate about the sexual specificity of sex hormones was also extended to the terminology and classification of sex hormones.

In the 1930s, many scientists expressed discontent with the terminology and classification of sex hormones, referring to these substances as "so-called" female sex hormones or simply putting the labels between parentheses. In this debate the Amsterdam School seems to have played an important role. They repeatedly criticized the use of the names "male" and "female" sex hormones. In the Dutch journal *Het Chemisch Weekblad* John Freud concluded in 1936:

> On purpose we avoid classification in terms of male and female hormones. Maybe our laboratory has contributed the most to overthrowing

this classification, since it has been proven experimentally that the oestrogenic substances of the male and the comb-growth stimulating substances of the female have certain functions and are found in the urine of both sexes.

(J. Freud 1936)

The Amsterdam School even expressed their doubts about whether these substances should be classified as sex hormones:

These substances are historically named sex hormones not because they are very important for sexual development, but merely because the changes these substances bring about in the organism can be observed with rather crude techniques of observation.

(J. Freud 1936)

In addition to the Dutch scientists, the British physiologist Vladimir Korenchevsky was also rather averse to the classification of male and female sex hormones; and both groups proposed other classifications (Korenchevsky and Hall 1938: 998). Korenchevsky and his colleagues proposed a classification of sex hormones into three groups: purely male and female hormones (active only in male or female organisms), partially bisexual hormones (hormones with chiefly male or female properties), and true bisexual hormones (active in both sexes) (Korenchevsky *et al.* 1937).[23]

Laqueur's group suggested that these substances might better be classified as catalysts, thus accommodating the wide variety of their functions (J. Freud 1936: 12). From a chemical perspective, they even proposed abandoning the entire concept of sex hormones:

If we understand the hormones as catalysts for certain chemical conversions in cells, it would be easier to imagine the manifold activities of each hormonal substance ... maybe the greatest discovery in the area of sex hormones will be the detection of the chemical conversions in the cells which are caused by steroids with certain structural qualities. Then the empirical concept of sex hormones will disappear and a part of biology will definitely pass into the property of biochemistry.

(J. Freud 1936: 12–14)

As against this proposal, the zoologist Frank Lillie intended to adhere to the old names:

The great advances that have been made and consolidated especially in the chemistry and chemical relationships of the male and female sex hormones and in the study of the relations between gonads and hypophysis and of the gonadotropic hormones have served to complicate rather than to simplify our conceptions of the mechanisms of control of sexual characteristics. It seems inadvisable to include in a biological introduction the newer chemical terminology. The old terms male and female sex hormones carry the implication of control of sexual characteristics and represent conceptions that would be valid whatever the outcome of further chemical and physiological analysis.

(Lillie 1939: 6)

The debate about the terminology and classification of sex hormones makes it clear how the different professional backgrounds of the disciplines involved in hormonal research led to a different conceptualization of sex hormones. Biochemists assigned meanings to their objects of study that were different from those of biologists. The hormone of the biochemist is in many respects quite different from the hormone of the biologists. From the chemical perspective, hormones were conceptualized as catalysts: chemical substances, sexually unspecific in origin and function, exerting manifold activities in the organism, instead of being primarily sex agents. From the biological perspective, hormones were conceptualized as sexually specific agents, controlling sexual characteristics.

What exactly happened to these different interpretations? Which interpretation of hormones became accepted as the dominant conceptualization of sex hormones? Although the chemical interpretation – emphasizing the resemblance of male and female sex hormones and the possibility of conversion from one to the other – did provoke confusion in the field of sex endocrinology, the prediction of the Amsterdam School was not fulfilled: the biological concept of sex hormones did not disappear. In the 1930s, we see the frequent use of a more specialized, technical terminology for sex hormones. Female sex hormones became known as estrin and estrogen (as a collective noun). For the male sex hormone the names androsterone and testosterone as specialized terms, and androgens as a collective term, became more frequently used. This new terminology did not, however, replace the old terms of female and male sex hormones.[24] Although scientists abandoned the concept of sexual specificity, the terminology was not adjusted to this change in conceptualization. The concept of sex hormones thus showed its robustness under major changes in theory, allowing talk of sex hormones to continue unabated, even though new properties were being ascribed to the hormones. From the 1930s until recently, the names male and female sex hormones have been kept in current use, both inside and outside the scientific community.[25] In this respect the biological perspective overruled the chemical perspective.

This outcome illustrates the strength of the tradition of biologists in the young field of sex endocrinology. The biologists had established a much longer tradition in the field than the biochemists, who were after all newcomers in the field. This does not mean that biologists can be portrayed as the "winners" of the debate. Both biochemists and biologists adjusted their interpretations of the concept of sex hormones: biologists adjusted their original interpretation of sex hormones as substances sexually specific in origin and function; while biochemists dropped their interpretation of hormones as catalysts. The interpretation that finally came to dominate the field may thus be considered as the result of a compromise between biologists and biochemists.

ON MASCULINE WOMEN AND FEMININE MEN

In the previous sections we have seen how sex endocrinologists gradually transformed the prescientific idea of a sexual duality located in the gonads into a conceptualization of sex that became more and more remote from common-sense opinions about sex and the body. In the paradigm of sex endocrinology, the essence of femininity and masculinity was no longer located primarily in the gonads, but extended to the adrenals. Moreover, the control of sexual characteristics was not resticted to the gonads but was conceptualized as a complex feedback system between the gonads and the brain. This conceptualization meant a definitive break with common-sense opinions that the essence of femininity and masculinity was located in the gonads, a cultural notion that could be traced back to early civilization. That sex endocrinologists were aware of this break is shown in the following quotation from *The Sex Complex: A Study of the Relationship of the Internal Secretions to the Female Characteristics and Functions in Health and Disease*:

> It used to be thought that a woman is a woman because of her ovaries alone. As we shall see later, there are many individuals with ovaries who are not women in the strict sense of the word and many with testes who are really feminine in many other respects.
>
> (Bell 1916: 5)

The major question that emerges now is: what were the consequences of this new approach to the study of the human body? What was the impact of the introduction of the concept of sex hormones on the conceptualization of sex? A comparison with other fields in the life sciences reveals that the introduction of sex hormones generated a revolutionary change in the study of sex. For the first time in the history of the life sciences, sex was formulated in terms of chemical substances in addition to bodily structures such as organs or cells. Prior to the emergence of sex endocrinology, the study of sex differences had been traditionally the domain of anatomists and physiologists. In the sixteenth century, only the organs directly related to sexuality and reproduction were sexualized. In the course of the eighteenth century, the study of sex differences became a priority in scientific research. Since then, the sexualization of the body has been extended to anatomical structures not related to sexuality and reproduction, such as the skeleton, the blood and the brain.[26]

The introduction of the concept of sex hormones as chemical messengers controlling masculinity and femininity meant a shift in the conceptualization of sex from an anatomical entity to a chemical agency. Instead of identifying which organ was considered as the seat of femininity and masculinity, sex endocrinologists looked for the causal mechanism which regulates the development of the organism either into a male or a female. With the emergence of sex endocrinology and genetics the study of sex differences focussed on the causality rather than on the identification of sex. Sex endocrinologists claimed to provide the basic mechanism of sexual differentiation, a knowledge considered far more fundamental to a thorough understanding of sex than that which anatomists had provided.

The introduction of the concept of sex hormones not only meant a shift in the study of sex away from an anatomical identification of the body to a causal explanation of sexual differentiation, but also entailed another major change in the study of sex. Instead of locating the essence of femininity or masculinity in specific organs, as the anatomists had done, sex endocrinologists introduced a quantitative theory of sex and the body. The idea that each sex could be characterized by its own sex hormone was transformed into the idea of relative sexual specificity. Sex endocrinologists suggested that, although female sex hormones were more important for women (especially during pregnancy) than for men, their potency was the same in both sexes. Male sex hormones were thought to be of greater importance for the internal and external phenotype of men, but this was regarded as only a difference of degree. In *The Annual Review of Physiology* published in 1939, the American physiologist Herbert Evans postulated this theory as follows:

> It would appear that maleness or femaleness cannot be looked upon as implying the presence of one hormone and the absence of the other, but that differences in the absolute and especially relative amounts of these two kinds of substances may be expected to characterize each sex and, though much has been learned, it is only fair to state that these differences are still incompletely known.
>
> (Evans 1939: 578)

Or as Robert Frank suggested:

> The explanation naturally suggesting itself is in favor of the theory of a quantitative and fluid transition from male to female.
>
> (Frank 1929: 115)

With this quantitative theory, the endocrinologists introduced a new conceptualization of sex. In the earlier anatomical definition of sex individuals could be classified into two, or actually three, categories: on the basis of the type of sexual organs an individual was categorized as male or female, and in cases where an individual possessed the sexual organs of both sexes, as a hermaphrodite. However, with the new concept of relative sexual specificity endocrinologists constructed a biological foundation for a definition of sex in which an individual could be classified in many categories varying from "a virile to effeminate male" or from "a masculine to a feminine female," as Robert Frank described it. Laqueur's group described this conceptualization of sex in 1928 as follows:

> The occurrence of the female hormone in the male body gives rise to many fantastic reflections. . . . It is now proved that in each man there is something present that is inherent in the female sex. Whether we will succeed in determining the individual ratio of each man, in terms of a given percentage femininity, we don't know.
>
> (Borchardt *et al.* 1928: 1,028)

Other scientists joked, privately, that the new biochemistry meant the end of sex differences: "there but for one hydroxyl group go I" (Long Hall 1976: 20).

The new model of sex in which sex differences are ascribed to hormones as chemical messengers of masculinity and femininity, agents that are present in female as well as male bodies, made possible a revolutionary change in the biological definition of sex. The model suggested that, chemically speaking, all organisms are both male and female. Sex could now be conceptualized in terms of male/masculine and female/feminine, with the elements of these two pairs no longer considered *a priori* as exclusive. In this model, an anatomical male could possess feminine characteristics controlled by female sex hormones, while an anatomical female could have masculine characteristics regulated by male sex hormones.

This hormonal model of sex provided the life sciences with a model to explain the "masculine characteristics" in the female body and vice versa. In obstetric science, for example, the hormonal model was used in the 1930s to substantiate the classification of female pelves into "masculine" and "feminine" types.[27] Physicians and clinicians used the quantitative model of sex to account for the purportedly feminine character of homosexual men. In the next chapter we shall see how sex endocrinologists introduced diagnostic tests to measure the degree of femininity and masculinity in the human body.

This shift in thinking was found in other fields of science as well. After 1925, the concepts of masculinity and femininity became the central focus of research in psychology, next to the study of sex differences (Lewin 1984: 158). And similarly in anthropology: in 1935, Margaret Mead wrote her classic work *Sex and Temperament* in which she postulated the idea that masculinity and femininity are randomly distributed between the sexes by nature but are assigned to only one sex by society (Lewin 1984: 166).

endocrinology depends
on sex hormones . . .

CONCLUSIONS

Evaluating this case study, we may conclude that prescientific ideas are a major factor in structuring scientific development. The early history of sex endocrinology illustrates in the first place how the prescientific idea of a sexual duality located in the gonads functioned as a major guideline structuring the development of endocrinological research. At the beginning of each new line of research, scientists proposed hypotheses corresponding to the cultural notion of sexual duality. In research on the origin as well as on the function of sex hormones, hypotheses were directed by this assumption, thus producing friction between expectations and experimental data.

How science gives meaning to sex differences is thus partly shaped by cultural notions of masculinity and femininity. Scientists use cultural notions as one of their cognitive resources. This conclusion is in line with feminists' claims that the development of knowledge is shaped by cultural norms about women and men. This does not imply that science leaves these cultural notions unchanged, as is often assumed in feminist studies. Scientists not only use cultural ideas as cognitive resources, but also actively modify these notions. This study showed how sex endocrinologists incorporated the cultural notion of a sexual duality located in the gonads, and subsequently transformed this notion into a model of sex differences that inplied a drastic change in the conceptualization of sex differences.

In this respect, the story of sex hormones deviates from Fleck's story of syphilis. Fleck concluded that, despite the different cognitive approaches, scientists eventually maintained the cultural notions about syphilis. He described the development of the Wasserman test in terms of the ultimate realization of the prescientific idea of syphilis as bad blood (Belt and Gremmen 1988). The concept of sex hormones, however, is not simply a realization of prescientific ideas. In the case of sex hormones, differences in disciplinary styles contributed to a drastic change in the cultural notion of sexual duality. I described how biochemists approached the study of sex hormones from a perspective different from that of biologists and gynecologists. The hormone of the biochemist differed from the hormone of the biologist and the gynecologist. Gynecologists (studying dysfunctions of organs) and biologists (studying the physiological development of the organism) shared a common interest in functions. Biochemists (focusing mainly on chemical structures) were devoted to the study of structures rather than functions. Consequently, the disciplines gave different interpretations to the function of sex hormones, and they opted for different forms of classification and naming. Biochemists saw the object of their research in terms of catalysts: chemical substances, sexually unspecific in origin and function, inducing chemical conversions in the cells, thus emphasizing the manifold activities of the substances as major characteristics of sex hormones. Gynecologists and biologists interpreted their object of study as sex hormones: substances sexually specific in origin and function, thus highlighting as a major characteristic the function of these substances in the sexual development of the organism. Sex hormones thus embody the ideas and interests of different disciplinary traditions. This multidisciplinary context accounts for the changes that took place in the conceptualization of sex differences, a process in which the prescientific idea of a sexual duality located in the gonads became transformed into a chemical model of sex that enabled the construction of new meanings and practices that became attached to the human body.

This chapter focused primarily on the ideas and conceptual frameworks of sex endocrinologists. Science, however, is not just ideas. Scientists use other powerful tools in knowledge production. In the next chapter we focus more closely on one specific tool: the experiment.

3 The measuring of sex hormones

The most revolutionary aspect of the concept of sex hormones is the idea that sex is not restricted to the world of living organisms. Since the early decades of the twentieth century even chemicals have had a sex of their own. In their journals and textbooks scientists discuss male sex hormones, female sex hormones and heterosexual hormones as a reality that simply exists in nature. I became really intrigued by this image of sex hormones. Even today the naturalistic reality of sex hormones is often taken for granted, as is exemplified in Camille Paglia's *Sexual Personae*:

> Lust and aggression are fused in male hormones. Anyone who doubts this has probably never spent much time around horses.
>
> (Paglia 1991: 24)

This uncritical acceptance of female and male sex hormones as natural facts is related to the positivistic notion that science describes the world as it is. Constructivist approaches in science studies, however, brought the critical awareness that scientists do not describe reality, but that they create realities. This approach is most vividly portrayed in Ian Hacking's (1986) *Representing and Intervening* in which he describes the laboratory sciences in terms of their power to create artefacts: phenomena that did not exist prior to the intervention of laboratory scientists. In the words of Hacking:

> Laboratory science ... involves the creation of phenomena: the purification and stabilization of phenomena that cannot exist in pure condition in the universe ... In the laboratory, phenomena can be maintained, be recalled if interesting, be forgotten, or be transformed in ready made transferable technologies. This idea of purification, creation, and regulation of phenomena (including the world we live in) implies thinking and theorizing over the material reality. In addition, it implies interaction with reality, and, in a non-metaphorical sense, the recreation of this reality. What I address here is not the construction of facts as facts (metaphorically speaking), but the calling into existence of events and regularities.
>
> (Hacking 1989: 19–20)

In this constructivist approach sex hormones do not simply exist in nature, they are literally created by laboratory scientists. Or to quote Hacking again:

> We did not find sex hormones somewhere in a lost corner, like a desert island lost in the mist. We ourselves called sex hormones into existence.
>
> (Hacking 1989: 21)

What Hacking describes here is precisely what science makes so powerful: its capacity to create new things and new worlds. By doing this, laboratory sciences establish a material authority that is very dominant in our present culture. The new science of sex endocrinology established its material authority by transforming the theoretical concept of sex hormones into material realities: chemical substances with a sex of their own. By selecting specific methods of testing, scientists defined which substances they would label as "male" or "female."

The role of experiments in sex endocrinology did not, however, remain restricted to the laboratory. Sex endocrinologists enhanced their material authority by transferring the test methods developed in the laboratory to the clinic. Reconstructing the role of experiments in sex endocrinology, this chapter describes how disciplinary styles interact with laboratory practices, thus structuring the manner in which scientists give meaning to sex and the body, in both the laboratory and the clinic. In the process of testing, sex endocrinologists became more and more removed from common-sense opinions about sex and reshaped the meanings of masculinity and femininity.

TESTS FOR FEMALE SEX HORMONES

In *The Female Sex Hormone* (1929) Robert Frank suggested: "The female principle which we call the female sex hormone is widely distributed throughout the vegetable and animal kingdom." Frank described the presence of the "female principle" in a wide variety of substances, not only originating from animals and not even restricted to the females of the species. The list in this first handbook on female sex hormones included substances such as yeast, the buds of willows, potatoes, sugar beet, rice, ovaries and placenta, the body fluids of males such as blood, urine and bile, and even testes (Frank 1929: 109).

How did scientists decide which substances they would classify as female sex hormones? In the early decades of the twentieth century scientists suggested that the label "female" should be attached to substances that could restore the organism after removal of the ovaries. This criterion enabled researchers to choose from a whole series of suitable testing methods. In theory, any character or function that changed in the organism after the removal of the ovaries, and could be restored to its original state by the administration of preparations which were expected to contain the "female principle," could serve the purpose of a bio-assay for female sex hormone (Frank 1929: 887). Prior research on the removal of the ovaries had already provided the requisite knowledge as to which functions or characteristics were affected by ovariectomy.

In the early years scientists largely agreed which substances were suitable to work with. Following the paradigm which considered the ovaries as the seat of femininity, they used extracts prepared from ovaries. There existed, however, less agreement about the test methods. Analysis of textbooks and journals of the 1920s shows that scientists applied a wide range of biological assays in deciding which substances they would label as female sex hormones. Each discipline seems to have adopted its own specific test. In the early studies, gynecologists in Paris and Vienna used the growth of the uterus – or more precisely the increased weight of the uterus in ovariectomized rabbits after administration of ovarian extracts – as a decisive criterion for the labeling of substances as female sex hormones (Gustavson 1939: 887). The choice of this test can be understood in terms of the tradition in the life sciences of considering the uterus as the female organ *par excellence*. Moreover, gynecologists preferred this test because of their professional interest in pregnancy. In addition to using this biological assay method, gynecologists also performed clinical trials in which ovarian preparations were evaluated for use in the treatment of various kinds of diseases associated with dysfunction of the ovaries.

In contrast to gynecologists, laboratory scientists introduced test methods based on a wider variety of functions and characteristics. Physiologists and zoologists tested ovarian preparations on the feathers of domestic fowl; the growth of mammary rudiments in male mice; the growth of the vulva and the mammary glands in infantile female rats; and muscular activity, basal metabolism, and the levels of calcium and sugar in blood, both in mice and in women (Frank 1929: 109). The fact that physiologists opted for a wider variety of tests than did gynecologists can be understood in the context of the tradition of their discipline, which studied the physiology of the animal organism in all its aspects. The different tests served different purposes. The feathers test, for instance, was used primarily to study the duration of the action of ovarian preparations. This bio-assay was considered a rather convenient test, because the administration of ovarian extracts left a continuous and permanent record on the feathers instead of merely being reflected in the status of their growth at a particular time, as was the case in the uterus test (Parkes 1985: 515). The test involving the growth of mammary rudiments in male mice was used as an indicator for very small amounts of ovarian preparations (Allen *et al.* 1939: 515).

Behavioral tests were also introduced, particularly by psychologists involved in the study of sex hormones. William C. Young, an animal psychologist at the University of Chicago, used reproductive behavior as a specific test for female sex hormones. Studies of reproductive behavior in animals had indicated that among the lower mammals, which include species frequently used in the laboratory such as guinea-pigs, rats and mice, the females usually mate only during a specific period, called estrus. Experiments indicated that these periods of sexual activity disappeared after ovariectomy, but could be restored by injections of ovarian preparations (Allen *et al.* 1939: 503). This behavioral test procedure was applied only in the early studies of sex hormones.[1]

The laboratory scientists and the gynecologists, however, could not agree about which test to accept as a decisive proof that an ovarian extract contained the "female principle." The laboratory scientists criticized the gynecologists for testing ovarian preparations in the clinic before their physiological and pharmacological effects had been determined. The biological test method developed by the gynecologists (the uterus test) was also criticized by laboratory scientists as inadequate (Borell 1985).[2] This dispute between gynecologists and laboratory scientists took place in the context of a growing need on the part of the pharmaceutical industry to improve the quality of its ovarian products. Gynecologists had claimed that the powders and pills available from the drug trade did not contain any active ovarian substance. In 1929 Frank warned his colleagues of the poor quality of these products:

> commercial extracts now placed upon the market show a woeful lack of potency and rapid deterioration. Unpleasant local reactions may arise at the site of injection. The prices of these pharmaceutical preparations are prohibitive. Consequently I warn against their general use until better products are at our disposal.
>
> (Frank 1929: 297)

Actually, skepticism about the quality of commercial ovarian products was the very reason why many gynecologists (e.g., the German gynecologist Bernhard Zondek) became involved in research on ovarian preparations.[3] This criticism emanating from the gynecological community was part of a growing professional concern about the quality of all types of drugs (Starr 1982: 131–132). Consequently, the pharmaceutical industry also became interested in biological test procedures that could confirm the quality of its products.

The dispute over the appropriate methods of assaying sex hormones was part of a more general struggle between laboratory scientists and clinicians, which can be seen as characteristic of this period in medical history. The early decades of the twentieth century were marked by the growing professionalization of the sciences, a process in which laboratory scientists presented themselves as the dominant professionals among those, including clinicians, who were concerned with natural phenomena. By emphasizing the superiority of physiological methods over therapeutic test methods, laboratory scientists claimed the position of experts on tests, thus defining the demarcation lines of their own profession (Borell 1985: 4,11,18).

In 1923, laboratory scientists introduced a new test method that in their opinion was much better than the prevailing methods for evaluating ovarian preparations. Two American scientists, Edgar Allen, a professor of anatomy at the Yale University School of Medicine, and Edward Doisy, a professor of biochemistry at the Medical School of the University of St Louis, introduced the vaginal smear test, which was based on cyclic changes in the epithelial cells of the vagina considered characteristic of estrus. In the 1920s, some gynecologists and pharmaceutical manufacturers started to apply this test in their research.

Laboratory scientists used other strategies as well to establish their position as experts in the growing field of sex endocrinology. Even more important than introducing new tests was their role in setting standards to reduce complexities in a field that was becoming increasingly complex. By the end of the 1920s, there existed a bewildering variety of test methods, since every new group that became involved in research on sex hormones introduced new assays. Laboratory scientists tried to handle these complexities by setting standards for tests and terminology. The need for standardization in general was strengthened by the difficulties that had been experienced by physicians, the public health services, and pharmaceutical manufacturers due to the existence of a variety of different units for expressing the potency of one and the same drug. The situation had been particularly troublesome during the First World War. As a result, the Health Organisation of the League of Nations initiated a series of international conferences to establish international agreement on biological standardization in various fields, including the research and development of sex hormones (Gautier 1935). British laboratory scientists played a major role in this process of standardization. The National Institute for Medical Research in London had at its disposal a special Department of Biological Standards, charged with establishing international biological standards for drugs, hormones and vitamins (Hartley 1936). Two conferences were organized for the standardization of sex hormones, both chaired by Henry Dale, the director of the National Institute for Medical Research. These conferences provided the first occasion for international discussion in the emerging field of sex hormones research. Physiologists and biochemists from Britain, the United States, France, Germany, Switzerland and The Netherlands participated in the standardization conferences and came to an agreement on standard tests, a common terminology and the development of biological standards (Dale 1935a; 1935b).

The first Conference on the Standardization of Sex Hormones, in 1932, settled the question of which biological test was most appropriate for labeling substances as female sex hormones. The vaginal smear test was accepted as the standard test for these substances, which were now called "oestrus-producing hormones." The conference agreed

> that by the term "specific oestrus-producing activity" is to be understood the power of producing, in the adult female animal completely deprived of its ovaries, an accurately recognizable degree of the changes characteristic of normal oestrus. For the present, the only such change regarded by the Conference as providing a suitable basis for quantitative determination of activity in comparison with the standard preparation is the series of changes in the cellular contents of the vaginal secretion of the rat or mouse.
>
> (Dale 1935a: 124)

In this manner, laboratory scientists reduced the complexities of hormonal research. The choice of one specific test method as a standard test simplified their experimental practice. The use of a standard test enabled scientists to compare their experimental data with their colleagues' experiments. At the same time, the selection of one specific test also restricted the broad scope of hormonal research. In 1936, Dutch scientists criticized what they called the "unitary school" in sex endocrinology, suggesting that the search for suitable test methods led scientists to neglect the other biological functions of sex hormones.[4]

In this process of standardization, the laboratory scientists, and not the gynecologists, determined which test was accepted as the standard test for female sex hormones. With the development of the vaginal smear test, laboratory scientists provided the other groups in the field with the techniques required to improve the quality of hormone preparations. Dutch laboratory scientists evaluated the introduction of the vaginal smear test as follows: "The work of Allen and Doisy enables us to replace vague concepts and general reflections by measure and number" (E. Laqueur *et al.* 1927a: 2,077). The activity of ovarian preparations was expressed in animal units, referring to the quantity required to restore estrus changes in the vagina of ovariectomized animals, a practice which showed a remarkable difference in terminology between Europe and the USA. Because European scientists usually experimented with mice and American scientists worked only with rats, "the female principle" was expressed in mouse or rat units, according to which side of the ocean one was on (Dale 1935b).

Although the first standardization conference reduced some of the complexities of the field, scientists soon faced other complexities. We saw in Chapter 2 how scientists initially opted for the existence of just one single female sex hormone. It was in the process of testing substances isolated from the ovaries that scientists gradually abandoned the "one hormone" doctrine. This meant that scientists had to decide again about standardization problems. Three years after the first conference took place, the Second Conference on the Standardization of Sex Hormones

(1935) was organized to discuss the terminology and standard tests for the "second" female sex hormone. At this conference scientists accepted the name "progesterone" for common use in scientific literature. The test on "the proliferation of the endometrium (uterus tissue) of the rabbit," first introduced by the British anatomist George Corner, became accepted as the standard test for progesterone (Dale 1935b).

In the 1910s and 1920s, the measuring of female sex hormones was solely in the hands of biologists and gynecologists. This situation changed drastically in the late 1920s. As a result of the introduction of urine as a research material, chemical methods of analysis came to be of greater importance, and consequently the new discipline of biochemistry became more and more involved in research concerning sex hormones.[5] Biochemists devoted their energies to the chemical isolation and identification of sex hormones.

This change in focus from biological to chemical methods was part of a general emphasis on chemical determinations in the process of standardization. The chairman of the standardization conferences on sex hormones, Sir Henry Dale, expressed this preference for chemical methods in 1935 as follows:

> It may be further recognised that biological methods of comparative assay, with their inherent limitations of accuracy and their heavy cost in material and skill, should be replaced by chemical determinations, whenever these can be made with as great accuracy and specificity as those based on animal tests. It may be hoped that, as knowledge of the biological important principles increases, remedies which still, with our present knowledge, can only be standardised by biological methods may pass, one by one, into the class in which chemical analysis will supersede biological standardisation.
>
> (Dale 1935b: 621)

After the chemical isolation and identification of the sex hormones in the 1930s, the labeling of substances as female sex hormones was no longer defined primarily by biological tests. Researchers were now able to attach the label "female" to ovarian and urine preparations following the analysis of their chemical structures. In the early 1930s, Laqueur's research group was the first to apply a chemical test procedure for female sex hormones, consisting of a color reaction for the quantitative determination of these substances (Walsh 1985: 12). Chemical test procedures, however, did not completely replace biological tests. Biological assays remained in use as devices to control the quality of chemically manufactured hormone preparations (J. Freud 1938: 1,667).

TESTS FOR MALE SEX HORMONES

In the measuring of female sex hormones it is obvious that the preferences for specific tests are specific to various disciplines. But what about the measuring of male sex hormones? How did scientists attach the label "male" to substances?

Using a logic similar to that used in the study of female sex hormones, scientists decided that the label "male sex hormone" should be attached to substances that could induce the recovery of the organism after removal of the testes. In theory, any characteristic that changed following castration was considered suitable as an assay. Research on male sex hormones differed from the study of female sex hormones, in that the development of tests for male sex hormones was the exclusive field of laboratory researchers, primarily physiologists and zoologists, some animal psychologists, and later biochemists. One of the first tests for male sex hormones was comb growth in castrated roosters: the comb test, which has a long history. The first report describing the effect of the removal of testes on comb growth was published as early as 1849 by the German physiologist Berthold, and is generally considered by endocrinologists to be "the first proof of endocrinological function as we know it today" (Beach 1981: 328). The Amsterdam School described this test in its essentials:

> The rooster wears a comb, which is, so to speak, the flag that is hoisted to announce the presence of his testes to the hens. On removal of the testes the flag is lowered: the comb atrophies and the rooster has become a capon.
>
> (Tausk 1978: 54)

In addition to the comb test, physiologists applied assays based on changes in fat deposits, body length and weight, and hair growth, in rats and guinea-pigs. The variety of tests illustrates the interest of physiologists in all aspects of the physiology of animal organisms. As in testing for female sex hormone, animal behavioral tests were also introduced, specifically tests that involved mating behavior (Beach 1981: 335). The chemical isolation and identification of male sex hormone in the 1930s enabled scientists to attach the label "male" to hormonal preparations following the analysis of their chemical structures. In contrast to female sex hormones, biochemists did not develop color reaction tests.

In the 1930s the comb test was the one most widely used. This testing method was accepted as the standard test for male sex hormones in 1935 at the Second Conference on Standardization of Sex Hormones in London. Consequently, the activity of testes preparations was expressed in rooster or capon units. Remarkably, the development of tests for male sex hormones involved less debate than did the development of tests for female sex hormones. As we have seen, the debate over the test procedure

for female sex hormones emerged from criticism of the quality of commercial ovarian preparations, expressed particularly by gynecologists. The
absence of such a debate about male sex hormones reflects a lack of
professional concern with the quality of male hormone preparations by
clinicians.

DISCIPLINARY STYLES AND INSTRUMENTAL INCENTIVES

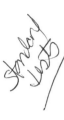

Evaluating the experimental practice of hormone research, we may conclude that disciplinary styles are an important factor in structuring the
laboratory activities of scientists. In the study of sex hormones, each
discipline opted for a specific type of test. Obviously, scientists have
specific disciplinary interests with regard to certain test methods. The
choice of standard tests can therefore also be understood in terms of the
influx of disciplines in a particular episode in the study of sex hormones.
For female sex hormones, the uterus test (introduced by gynecologists)
was supplemented by a whole series of tests from the moment that
laboratory scientists (and physiologists in particular) became involved in
the study of sex hormones. In the ultimate choice of a standard test, the
laboratory scientists – and not the gynecologists – were the leading
experts. With the influx of the biochemists, chemical testing methods
began to be used in the study of sex hormones.

Not only did disciplinary styles structure the choice of specific testing
methods, but also the aims of the tests were discipline- and actor-specific.
Throughout the years, the test methods have served different purposes in
the study of sex hormones. Biologists as well as gynecologists used tests
for two purposes: as a specific tool for sex labeling and as a tool to
investigate the function of sex hormones. The pharmaceutical industry
applied test methods merely to control the quality of hormone preparations. The biochemists used tests in order to isolate, identify and finally
synthesize sex hormones. Biochemists made sex hormones into substances
independent from the biological test methods in which they were shaped.

Disciplinary perspectives are thus a major factor in structuring the
activities in the laboratory. Scientists operate according to the traditions
of their fields. But are disciplinary styles the only factor that guide scientists in their daily practice? A closer look at the history of the measuring
of sex hormones reveals that the actual choice of the test methods has
been the result of instrumental as much as disciplinary considerations.

In measuring female sex hormones, instrumental incentives played a
major role in the decision about which test would be considered most
appropriate. In Allen's *Sex and Internal Secretions*, Reuben G. Gustavson
(1939), a professor of chemistry at the University of Colorado, emphasized
the fact that, compared with the other tests, the vaginal smear test had the
advantage of being rapid and inexpensive. The uterus test and most other
test methods were based on time-consuming surgical interventions in

experimental animals, a rather expensive matter because each new experiment required the use of new animals (Frank 1929: 887).[6] In this respect the vaginal smear test was considered to be rather revolutionary, because it enabled researchers to infer what was happening in the internal reproductive organs without having to perform surgery. As mentioned above, this test procedure consisted of tracing cytological changes in the reproductive tract during the estrus cycle, changes that extended also to the lower part of the vagina (Corner 1965: 12). In early experiments, Charles Stockard and George Papanicolaou, both zoologists at Cornell Medical College in New York City, had suggested that these cyclic changes should cease upon removal of the ovary and could be restored in the ovariectomized animal by the injection of ovarian preparations (Moore and Price 1932: 893). The cytological changes of the vagina could thus be determined by examining smears of easily accessible cells under the microscope. The color reaction test introduced by the biochemists also became widely used because this method was at least as accurate and convenient as the biological assay method and was even less time-consuming.

The choice of test methods for male sex hormones shows a similar pattern. In addition to disciplinary styles, instrumental considerations were of major importance in structuring the measuring of male sex hormones. The wide range of tests introduced by physiologists (like change in fat deposition, body length and weight, and hair growth) were considered not very convenient for routine use. The major disadvantage of these tests was that these functions and characteristics did not respond rapidly to castration or hormone treatment. The comb test also had practical disadvantages. The very choice of this test was one of the reasons why research on male sex hormones did not become current as fast as research on female sex hormones. It can easily be imagined that the keeping of roosters is rather inconvenient, particularly since most laboratories at that time had only limited space. Despite this disadvantage, the comb test was considered to be a rather convenient assay method because the test animals could be used several times and changes in the size of the comb could be detected easily (Tausk 1932a: 50). The test procedure consisted of measuring comb size in castrated roosters before and after hormone treatment (Figure 3.1). Laqueur and his co-workers at the University of Amsterdam introduced a photographic method in which the silhouette of the comb was photographed and changes in the comb size could be easily recorded (Frank 1929: 807–808).

The practical disadvantages of these tests led American scientists to introduce other testing methods for male sex hormones. Carl Moore and Dorothy Price, both zoologists from Chicago, suggested that tests involving the reproductive accessory organs of male rats, mice and guinea-pigs were most practical, because the effects of testes preparations could be seen within a reasonable length of time. One of these tests was based on the growth of seminal vesicles in castrated mice and rats. The seminal

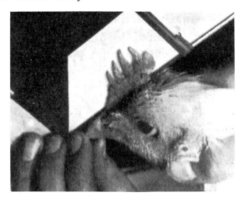

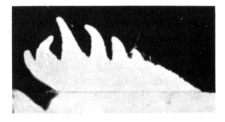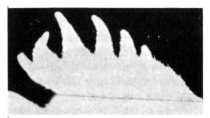

Figure 3.1 One of the standard tests for male sex hormones: the measurement of the comb size in castrated roosters before and after hormone treatment

vesicles test involved recording the weight of the seminal vesicles in castrated animals before and after administration of testes extracts (Koch 1939: 817). In addition to being a rather rapid test, this method also had the advantage that rats and mice could be kept much more easily than roosters.

In addition to the comb test, the seminal vesicles test became widely used and accepted as a standard test. In Allen's *Sex and Internal Secretions* male sex hormones are defined as "those substances, inducing the growth of the comb of castrated roosters as well as the growth of seminal vesicles in rats and mice" (Gustavson 1939: 877).

The actual choice of the standard biological test for sex hormones was thus also the result of instrumental incentives. In daily practice, scientists preferred those assays that were both easy to perform and inexpensive. Time-consuming tests, like assays using the feathers of poultry, were less suitable as daily routine procedures than tests on mice and rats, in which the effects of hormone administration could be detected within a short period of time. Obviously, these peculiarities of daily practices in the laboratory are a major factor in structuring the activities and choices of scientists.

With the choice of standard test methods, scientists defined the nature of what had to be considered as male or female sex hormones. It is

significant that in this process of sorting out the specific tests for sex
hormones, all functions and processes that were unrelated to sexual
characteristics and reproduction were dropped. The testing methods that
became accepted as standard tests for sex hormones were based not on
muscular activity or body weight, but on internal sexual organs (vagina
and seminal vesicles) and on a so-called secondary sexual characteristic
(the comb of the rooster). In this way, scientists attributed to the substances they had just isolated, and which they had named sex hormones,
the properties predicted by the biological paradigm in which sex hormones were defined as the chemical messengers of masculinity and femininity. Consequently, female sex hormones became related to female
sexual organs and male sex hormones to male sexual organs and characteristics.

Although the process of testing confirmed major assumptions underlying the conceptualization of sex hormones, at the same time it challenged other key assumptions about the "nature" of sex hormones. I
described in Chapter 2 how sex endocrinologists in their experiments
dropped the idea that there existed just one single hormone per sex. The
test methods also played a major role in rejecting the idea of the sexual
specificity of sex hormones, as described in Chapter 2. In the debate
about the sex specific origin and function of sex hormones, scientists
based their arguments largely on the results of their tests. Experiments
thus functioned as major devices in establishing as well as changing the
paradigm of sex endocrinology.

THE IMPACT OF LABORATORY TESTS ON MEDICAL PRACTICE

Use of the tests introduced by laboratory scientists was not restricted to
the laboratory. Sex endocrinologists involved in the study of sex hormones
transferred the tests from the laboratory to the clinic, thus enhancing
their material authority to a larger domain than just the laboratory. In
the 1930s, tests developed to measure the sex of substances were used
increasingly as diagnostic tools in the clinic. The next sections evaluate the
impact of the introduction of laboratory-based tests on medical practice.

Measuring disorders in the female body

The introduction of laboratory tests by sex endocrinologists had major
consequences for medical practice, particularly in the gynecological clinic.
As we saw in Chapter 2, gynecologists had entered the emerging field of
sex endocrinology mainly because of its promises of a better understanding and therefore greater control over the complex of disorders in women
frequently associated with the ovaries. The American gynecologist Robert
Frank described this interest of gynecologists in 1929 as follows:

The study of the female sex hormone ... has now reached the critical stage in which we may hope at any time to obtain a pure substance. Such an achievement will not only be another triumph for the physiologist, endocrinologist, and chemist, from the theoretical standpoint, but will carry with it many invaluable, practical results in the treatment of diseases of women.

(Frank 1929: 1)

The tests developed in the laboratory provided the gynecologists with a tool to measure female sex hormones in their female patients. Gynecologists expected that the excretion of hormones in urine indicated an abnormally high quantity of hormones in the female body which was considered as the cause of female disorders (E. Laqueur 1937). Robert Frank played a major role in transferring the laboratory tests to the women's clinic. In 1925 Frank was one of the first to investigate the presence of female sex hormone in the blood of female animals. This research facilitated Frank's move from the laboratory to the clinic, as he said. "Based upon these findings it was natural for me to study and investigate the human female" (Frank 1929: 177). One part of *The Female Sex Hormone* (1929) was devoted to "the biology, pharmacology and chemistry of the female sex hormone," and the other part solely to "the clinical investigations based on the female sex hormone blood test" (Figure 3.2).

The female sex hormone blood test consisted of injecting blood extract of female patients into test mice. Subsequently, the vaginal smear test was applied to determine the quantity of female sex hormone in the blood. The results of these tests were compared with the hormone blood level of "the normal woman," a standard that Frank derived from the average of blood tests in more than 500 women. The female sex hormone blood test was performed upon patients in whom abnormalities of the function of the ovaries were suspected (Frank 1929: 211). Frank applied this test for two general purposes. Based on his study of 500 patients Frank introduced a classification system of four types of women:

> On the basis of these studies, the patients examined have been divided into various groups which include women suffering from hypofunction of the ovaries, hyperfunction of the ovaries, major endocrine disturbances.... Most patients can be classified under 4 types, the normal feminine, the infantile, the eunuchoid, and the virile. In addition, more marked endocrine disturbances enable us to differentiate pituitary, thyroid, adrenal and gonadic types.

(Frank 1929: 295)

In addition to classification Frank used the female sex hormone blood test for the diagnosis of menstrual disorders (ascribed to hypofunction or hyperfunction of the ovaries), the diagnosis of pregnancy, and the differential diagnosis between pregnancy, amenorrhea (absence of menstrual

THE FEMALE SEX HORMONE

PART I

BIOLOGY, PHARMACOLOGY AND CHEMISTRY

PART II

CLINICAL INVESTIGATIONS BASED ON THE
FEMALE SEX HORMONE BLOOD TEST

BY

Robert T. Frank, A.M., M.D., F.A.C.S.

GYNECOLOGIST TO MOUNT SINAI HOSPITAL, NEW YORK

With 86 Illustrations and 36 Graphs

"*Propter secretiones internas totas, mulier est quod est*"

F. A. E. CREW [85]

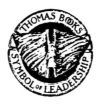

CHARLES C THOMAS · PUBLISHER

SPRINGFIELD, ILLINOIS   BALTIMORE, MARYLAND

MDCCCCXXIX

Figure 3.2 Title-page of *The Female Sex Hormone*, the first handbook on female sex hormones that appeared in 1929. *Source*: Frank (1929)

bleedings) and nonpregnant enlargements of the uterus. The test was also applied for sex determination "in the presence of malformation" (Frank 1929: 295).

In *The Female Sex Hormone* Frank propagated the use of the female sex hormone blood test to his colleagues, emphasizing the fact that this test could be easily performed in any hospital laboratory:

> the average hospital equipment and personnel is well able to perform this test as a routine just as the Wasserman test is performed in hospital laboratories. The space at our disposal has been limited to a single room. In this there are 25 rat cages in which 250 castrated mice can be kept for the test.
>
> (Frank 1929: 177)

Obviously, instrumental considerations are also a major factor in judging the usefulness of tests for the clinic.

The introduction of the vaginal smear test in the laboratory heralded yet another major change in the medical practice concerning the female body. Laboratory scientists focussed the attention of the medical profession on cellular changes in the vagina of the human female. In 1933 George Papanicolaou, one of the founding fathers of the vaginal smear test, suggested that this test could also be applied directly to women, indicating "potential and actual pathological changes in the cervix and uterus for diagnosis of cancerous and other abnormal conditions."[7] The introduction of the vaginal smear test in the clinic extended the medical intervention techniques from the uterus and the ovaries to the vagina. This technique provided gynecologists and physicians with a powerful new diagnostic tool to investigate their female patients. Since the 1930s, the vaginal smear technique (or "Pap smear" as this test came to be known in honor of Papanicolaou) has become increasingly applied as a potential indicator of menstrual disorders, and more recently as a diagnostic test in large-scale screening programs for cancer.

Measuring sex in homosexuals

Another way in which the hormonal tests came to be used in the clinic was in the treatment of homosexuals. In Chapter 2 we saw how clinicians expected that female sex hormones in male bodies caused disorders in masculinity. One of these "disorders" was homosexuality. The basic assumption underlying this hypothesis was that homosexual men were considered more or less "feminine," so that a connection with female sex hormones as the agents of femininity seemed likely. An analogous concept was developed for homosexual women, although most studies were performed on men (Meyer-Bahlburg 1984: 376).

In 1935 Clifford Wright, a general practitioner in Los Angeles, described this hormonal etiology of homosexuality:

All individuals are part male and part female, or bisexual, and this fact is substantiated by hormone assays in the urine. The urine of the normal man or woman shows the presence of hormones of both the male and female types. . . . In the normal male, the male hormone predominates; in the normal female, the female hormone predominates. This, in my opinion, is the cause of normal sex attraction. In the homosexual the dominance is reversed. In the man there is a predominance of the female element and in the homosexual woman a dominance of the male factor.

(Wright 1938: 249)

This conceptualization of homosexuality was perfectly in line with the then prevailing ideas about homosexuality. Many influential European sexologists working at the turn of the century, such as Richard von Krafft-Ebing, Havelock Ellis and Magnus Hirschfeld, asserted that homosexuality is determined by biological factors. Hirschfeld, one of the pioneers of equal rights for homosexuals, advocated the theory of intersexual stages (*Zwischenstufentheorie*), first introduced by a German lawyer, C.H. Uhlrichs, in the 1860s. In Hirschfeld's opinion, homosexuality was an intersexual stage between the poles of complete maleness and femaleness. In his theory, homosexual men and women were portrayed as physically male or female, but sexually and emotionally endowed with many characteristics of the other sex. Homosexuals were thus considered as hermaphrodites or a third sex.

The experiments of one of the pioneers in sex endocrinology, the Viennese anatomist Eugen Steinach, in which he claimed to have produced hermaphroditic animals by transplanting gonads from the other sex, fitted seamlessly into this theory of intersexual stages. Steinach referred to Hirschfeld when reflecting on his animal experiments: "Homosexuality can also be ascribed to the existence of a hermaphrodite pubertal gland, just as Hirschfeld rightly postulated when he talked about the congenital disposition of the homosexual" (Steinach 1916: 307). Steinach suggested that the testicles of homosexual males contained "deviated cells" which he called "F-cells" and which had a "feminizing or homosexual-making" effect (Lichtenstern 1920). Steinach's experiments did not remain restricted to animals. In 1916, he performed the first surgical operation in which he transplanted testicular tissue from a heterosexual man into a homosexual. Medical records indicate that at least eleven homosexual men underwent the "Steinach operation" between 1916 and 1921.[8] These experiments inextricably linked the discourse on homosexuality with the discourse on gender and launched the biomedical sciences' search for biological markers of femininity and masculinity in homosexuals.[9]

The introduction of the hormonal theory of homosexuality, and subsequently the introduction of tests to measure sex hormones in human bodies, provided clinicians with a means to replace gonadal transplant operations with hormone treatments. The new science of sex endocrinology defined homosexuality as an endocrine imbalance. In the 1930s, the laboratory tools developed to study sex hormones were applied to measure the "male" and "female" factor in homosexuals. Physicians tested urinary extracts of homosexual patients (mostly men) in their private practice or clinic. The vaginal smear test was applied to check for the presence of the "female element." The "male factor" was assayed with the comb test. The results of these tests were subsequently compared with the urinary hormone excretion rates of male and female sex hormones by "normal men and women" (read heterosexuals). The "normal" excretion of male sex hormones in men was set at an average of 25–45 capon units, whereas female sex hormone excretion should not exceed the norm of 12–14 mouse units (Wright 1938: 450). Homosexuality thus became expressed in terms of capon and mouse units.

With the use of these hormone assays the medical profession expected to distinguish "true congenital" homosexuals from "acquired" homosexuals. This idea is in accordance with the doctrine of nineteenth-century theoreticians that there existed two types of homosexuals: a hereditary or inborn form and an acquired or learned form. This doctrine assumed implicitly that the inborn homosexual could not be changed, whereas acquired homosexuality might be reversible (Money 1980: 7). Consequently, one of the two types of homosexuals could be "cured." Following the paradigm of sex endocrinology in which sex hormones were seen as the agents of masculinity and femininity, physicians expected that sex hormones could be used as specific drugs for the treatment of homosexuality. Soon after the first sex hormones were chemically identified and synthesized, homosexuals became increasingly treated with "sex appropriate" sex hormones to change their sexual orientation (Meyer-Bahlburg 1984: 376).

The homosexuality test was applied not only for medical reasons. Part of the physicians' practice consisted of court cases. Because homosexuality was considered a criminal act, the examination of the "true nature" of people suspected of homosexuality was of major importance (Wright 1938: 449). Sex endocrinologists now claimed to possess a scientific test to measure the "biological markers" of homosexuality.

The tests originally developed for laboratory research thus came to be used as diagnostic tests for medical and legal purposes, intervening into the lives of homosexual men for several decades. In the 1930s and 1940s, there were numerous treatments of male homosexuals with male sex hormones in the USA. In The Netherlands the hormonal treatment of homosexuality seems to have been practiced on a rather small scale. Publications in the *Nederlands Tijdschrift voor Geneeskunde* (*Dutch Journal for Medicine*) in the period between 1919 and 1949 do not address the hormone theory of homosexuality and describe homosexuality solely in terms of disorders in the sex glands.[10] In the archives of Organon the subject of homosexuality is addressed only twice. In 1934 Laqueur requested Organon to deliver *Menformon* (female sex hormone) free of charge to a general practitioner in order to investigate the effects of female sex hormones in a case involving female twins, one of whom was heterosexual and the other homosexual. Beyond a brief inquiry in 1935 following the results of this experiment, stating that Organon was very interested in this newly discovered area, the issue of hormone therapy in homosexuality was addressed only once more in 1936, when Laqueur inquired about medical literature on hormones and lesbianism. In its *Pocket Lexicon for Organ and Hormone Therapy* Organon included homosexuality as susceptible to hormonal therapy, but suggested that "for the time being, homosexuality can not be affected with any certainty" (Anonymous 1937).

REDEFINING MASCULINITY AND FEMININITY

The introduction of testing methods for sex hormones not only changed medical practices but also transformed the meanings science assigned to sex differences in different respects.

First, in the process of testing we see how scientists gradually became more and more remote from common-sense opinions and everyday language. In the early period of hormonal research, scientists still used concepts that were closely related to common-sense notions of masculinity and femininity. Based on their test methods, sex endocrinologists defined sex hormones as substances originating from ovaries and testes, a conceptualization which strongly resembles the prescientific idea of the ovaries and testes as the seat of femininity and masculinity. Entering more deeply into the laboratory, we encounter an increasingly specialized technical language and conceptualization of sex hormones. In their later experiments, gynecologists defined sex hormones as substances regulating the growth of the uterus. When biologists and chemists enter the field, we see a wide variety of statements about hormones with an increasing array of technical details:

1 female hormones induce the cornification of the epithelial cells of the vagina in ovariectomized mice
2 the extracts of bull testes induce the growth of the atrophic comb of the capon
3 male sex hormones are steroids, melting point 183.5–184.5°C, and are alkali labile
4 the molecular formula of testosterone is $C_{19}H_{28}O_2$.

This list of statements reveals how, in the process of testing, the culturally based definition of sex is gradually replaced with an increasingly technical account of sex and the body.

Second, in choosing specific test methods for sex hormones, scientists not only introduced a technical account of sex, but also specified the meanings they assigned to sex. In Chapter 2, we saw how sex endocrinologists gradually abandoned the original assumption that each sex could be recognized by its own sex hormone. Instead, sex endocrinologists introduced a quantitative theory of sex in which male and female sex hormones are present in both sexes. Men and women differ only in the relative amounts of their sex hormones. The introduction of tests for measuring sex hormones provided sex endocrinologists with the tools to specify this quantitative theory. Based on the female sex hormone blood test, gynecologists now suggested that men and women could be characterized by the specific nature of their hormone regulation, emphasizing the cyclic nature of female sex hormone production in women and the continuous, stable nature of male sex hormone production in men (Frank 1929: 113, 292). Sex endocrinology thus attached the quality of cyclicity to femininity, and stability to masculinity.

The emphasis on cyclicity is also reflected in the naming of one of the female sex hormones. One of the two types of female sex hormones was renamed "estrogens", thus referring to the specific test method for female sex hormones: the cyclic changes in the vagina characteristic of estrus, the period of sexual activity and fertility. By choosing the name estrogens, sex endocrinologists emphasized the cyclic nature of female reproductive function. Although cyclicity can have positive connotations (cyclicity means regularity) as well as negative connotations (cyclicity means instability), scientists emphasized the latter. The next quote from a Dutch gynecologist exemplifies how scientists associated femininity with lability:

> Throughout her entire life the woman is controlled by the rhythmic function of her ovaries, and the changing hormonal content of her blood causes a major psychological and bodily lability. For men such a problem does not exist. This is the reason why women are handicapped in their struggle for equality with men.
>
> (Snoo 1940: 3,940)

In Chapter 4, we shall see how the association of femininity with cyclicity also affected medical practice. This association has functioned as paradigmatic both in later studies and medical practice with respect to many different aspects of the female body. The emphasis on the cyclicity of female reproductive functions disclosed the possibility of medical intervention into the cyclic functions, like intervening into the length of the menstrual cycle by administering hormones.

Finally, the introduction of tests also created extensive changes in the sex labeling of physical features. In this process, sex endocrinologists redefined what had to be considered as male and female characteristics. The manner in which scientists redefined male and female characteristics is nicely illustrated in the *Handbuch der biologischen Arbeitsmethoden*, one of the first handbooks on biological research methods, published in 1938. In the chapter dealing with research techniques for male sex hormones, male characteristics are classified into three categories: physical characteristics, psychic characteristics and neutral characteristics (J. Freud 1938: 1,671). In the context of this study, the last category is of particular interest. Neutral characteristics are defined as those male or female features that do not change after castration or ovariectomy. With this premise endocrinologists actually redefined what should be considered as male or female characteristics. Physical features considered as typically male or female before endocrinology emerged were now considered as sex-neutral. For example, the feathers and spurs of domestic fowl, with striking differences between males and females, were no longer classified as male or female characteristics but as neutral features.

Other scientists argued, however, that these features should not be classified as sex neutral. Dutch and British scientists introduced a new classification of sex characteristics. In addition to male and female characteristics, they suggested using the categories of "negative masculine" and "negative feminine." In contrast to what endocrinologists had expected, the gaudy plumage of roosters seemed to be controlled not by male sex hormones but by female sex hormones. In domestic fowl, castration of the male had no effect on the feathers, whereas ovariectomy of the female resulted in the male type of feathering. Thus, in the terms of endocrinologists, a hen is hen-feathered because her "male" plumage is suppressed by the activity of female sex hormones (Callow and Parkes 1936: 7). Features like the plumage of roosters were now redefined as "negative feminine" characteristics (Jongh 1951: 20).

Hair growth on the heads of men confronted endocrinologists with similar problems. This hair growth was considered as a feature stimulated by male sex hormones. Consequently, hair growth was considered a typically masculine characteristic. Following this definition, the phenomenon that men usually lose their hair with increasing age could no longer be considered as masculine. Endocrinologists renamed this feature as "negative masculine." (Jongh 1951: 20).

Sex endocrinologists thus redefined the sex labeling of physical features. Following the basic criterion for sex hormones embodied in the biological tests, only those functions and characteristics whose development was stimulated by male or female sex hormones were still entitled to be labeled masculine of feminine. Features that were not controlled by sex hormones were considered as sexually neutral, whereas features whose development was suppressed by sex hormones were labeled as "negative masculine" or "negative feminine."

CONCLUSIONS

In this chapter we have seen how the new science of sex endocrinology established its material authority. By focussing on one specific feature in the laboratory, the experiment, we obtained a more detailed picture of the impact of laboratory science on meanings and practices concerning the human body. This episode also had major consequences for the relationships between the disciplines involved in hormone research. In times when the development of standard tests was central to the field, the relationships between the different disciplines changed drastically. I described in Chapter 2 how, in the early years, clinicians – mainly gynecologists and some physiologists involved in paramedical practices – dominated the field. Laboratory scientists – zoologists, physiologists and biochemists – did not enter the field before the 1910s. Initially, these different disciplines occupied equal positions in the networks that gradually emerged between clinicians and laboratory scientists.

In the 1920s, the tables were turned. The relationship between the clinicians and laboratory scientists changed from that of equal partners into one increasingly dominated by laboratory scientists. I described how laboratory scientists presented themselves as the dominant profession in hormone research. What they brought into the field was their expertise in developing testing methods, and introducing new techniques and methods for standardization. In this manner, laboratory scientists established their authority as experts on tests which were crucial in producing standardized hormone preparations and to reduce the complexities in the field. Laboratory scientists thus succeeded in establishing a strategic position in the networks with clinicians, as well as with the third group that became more and more interested in hormone research: the pharmaceutical entrepreneurs. Clinicians, as well as pharmaceutical companies, became dependent on the expertise of laboratory scientists.

The role of clinicians in the research networks changed from that of leading scientists to audiences. Laboratory scientists transferred the testing of sex hormones from the clinic to the laboratory. In this period, the laboratory became the center of research. The clinic now became an audience for the products of the laboratory. I described how laboratory scientists took something from the pioneering clinicians, that is their early experience in testing hormone preparations, and gave it back to them in the form of diagnostic tools for the clinic.

Pharmaceutical companies became dependent on laboratory scientists for the provision of the required biological assay techniques in order to manufacture standardized hormone products. Laboratory scientists transferred human beings, skills and apparatus from the laboratory to industry. In The Netherlands, for example, the personnel of Organon were trained in testing techniques at Laqueur's laboratory at the University of Amsterdam before they were employed as workers in the pharmaceutical firm. Those who had been directly involved in the preparation of hormonal products could be employed only with the permission of Laqueur. Laqueur also moved equipment from his laboratory in Amsterdam to Organon

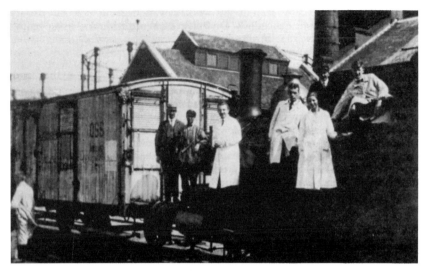

Figure 3.3 The instrumental equipment of Laqueur's laboratory arrives at the grounds of Organon in Oss, 1 August, 1923.
Source: Organon Archives

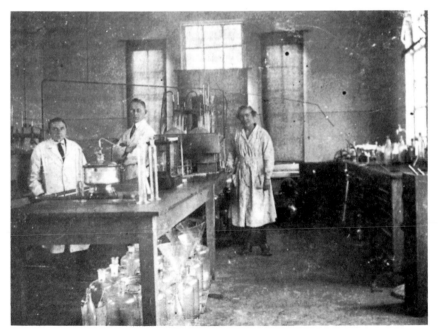

Figure 3.4 Organon's laboratory in 1923
Source: Organon Archives

in Oss to set up the pharmaceutical firm's first research laboratory (Figures 3.3 and 3.4).[11] In the next chapter I shall go into more detail about these relationships between laboratory scientists and pharmaceutical companies.

This episode of testing not only shaped the interrelationships of laboratory scientists, clinicians and pharmaceutical companies, but also was crucial in according knowledge claims about sex hormones a universal, context-independent character. Local laboratory practices became universalized by developing instruments, techniques and context-independent standards robust enough to survive outside the laboratory. Laboratory scientists provided the field of sex endocrinology with a means to lift local practices out of their specific contexts. The setting of standards of measurement played a major role in changing laboratory practices into practices that could be made to work elsewhere: the pharmaceutical company and the clinic. Test methods provided sex endocrinologists with the tools to transform the theoretical concept of sex hormones into standardized chemical substances that could exist apart from the laboratory conditions that shaped them. This transformation of sex hormones into material realities required yet another major tool: research materials. In the next chapter we shall follow the different groups involved in the study of sex hormones in their search for the tons of ovaries, testes and urine required in the making of sex hormones.

4 The making of sex hormones

In 1934, a cargo train arrived at the grounds of the Dutch pharmaceutical company Organon. This train did not carry any conventional cargo such as coal, or instrumental equipment, but a rather extraordinary load: thousands of liters of urine. In the Dutch countryside, horse owners could sell the liquid waste products of their mares for prices equal to the price of cows' milk. In the mean time, people living near the site of Organon complained about a very peculiar, unpleasant smell that penetrated their houses. Elsewhere in Europe and in the United States, scientists visited slaughterhouses to collect organic remains. In Britain, scientists ordered the delivery of a blue whale to their laboratories. What was happening? What connects these, at first sight, separate events? The collection, selling and transport of urine, the search for remains from slaughterhouses and the ordering of a whale were all aimed at the same goal: the production of sex hormones. The making of sex hormones into material realities required the availibility of tons of ovaries and testes, as well as millions of liters of urine.

In the previous chapter we saw how scientists used test methods to identify, isolate and finally to synthesize chemical substances which they labeled as male and female sex hormones. This chapter analyzes another major material condition for the creation of sex hormones: the role of research materials. The major location featuring in the previous chapters was the laboratory. In the making of sex hormones into chemicals, other settings became increasingly important in structuring the hormonal enterprise. In order to obtain the required research materials, scientists were largely dependent on arrangements with institutions outside the laboratory: the clinic and the pharmaceutical industry.

These arrangements highlight a very crucial feature in the development of scientific research. The production of scientific facts and artefacts obviously does not take place in isolated laboratories by individual scientists. Recent constructivist science studies hold that, to make science work, scientists have to leave their laboratories and create alliances with other relevant social groups. (Bijker 1993; Pinch and Bijker 1987) This chapter explores how scientists made sex hormones into artefacts. I describe how sex endocrinologists created networks with the pharmaceutical industry and the clinic in order to organize the material conditions necessary for their research. The deceptively simple question – which research materials did scientists use in the making of sex hormones? – thus leads us into a much more complex analysis of how science works. How do laboratory scientists, clinicians and pharmaceutical entrepreneurs come together as major groups in the hormonal endeavor? What type of alliances did they create? What bound them together? How did the subject of sex hormones evolve into a mutually shared topic of interest among laboratory scientists, clinicians and pharmaceutical companies?

To answer these questions, we follow the different groups involved in the making of sex hormones in their efforts to gain access to the required research materials, focussing particularly on Dutch sex endocrinologists. I describe how the accessibility of research materials affected both the character of the relationships between the laboratory, the clinic and the pharmaceutical company, and the strategic position of each group involved in these networks. The chapter proceeds to analyze how the access to research materials affected the research agenda in the emerging field of sex endocrinology. These materials were not just a resource, but functioned as carriers of knowledge claims, facilitating a situation in which the study of female sex hormones, and not male sex hormones, gradually developed into big science and big business.

GAINING ACCESS TO RESEARCH MATERIALS

The role of research materials in scientific research seems quite evident. Scientists need research materials in order to study their topics of interest. Day-to-day practices in the laboratory consist in large measure of obtaining and managing research materials. Problems in the supply of research materials might present major constraints to scientists' activities. If scientists do not manage to obtain the required materials, they simply cannot work. Research materials are thus an important practical resource for the production of knowledge.

Problems in gaining access to research materials seem to have been particularly manifest in the life sciences at the turn of the century. Scientific research in this period was characterized by a shift from descriptive, morphological approaches to experimental approaches. The new experimental approaches radically altered scientists' needs for research materials (Clarke 1987b). The need for new types of research materials is very evident in the field of sex endocrinology. Scientists entering this field had to have access to research materials not yet routinely used in the laboratory: ovaries and testes.

How did sex endocrinologists gain access to these rather unfamiliar materials? A perusal of the scientific literature reveals that the search for gonads was not easy. The reports of sex endocrinologists are filled with complaints about the scarcity of ovaries and testes. These complaints seem to have been particularly loud in the 1920s. What was happening at that time? By the 1920s, scientists were confronted with a specific handicap – namely, the problem of how to obtain adequate quantities of the research materials required for the preparation of gonadal extracts. Previous research had been focussed solely on the biological function of gonadal extracts. Relatively small amounts of raw material were required for these experiments. One kilogram of testes was sufficient to study the effects of gonadal extracts in the organism.

Prior to the 1920s, the groups involved in the study of sex hormones had no serious problems in obtaining access to the required research materials. Gynecologists obtained research materials from their own patients. Since the 1870s surgical operations for the removal of human ovaries had become common practice in gynecology, and consequently gynecologists had easy access to the research materials required for their experiments. Later, the placenta and animal ovaries were also used as research materials (Corner 1965: 4, 10). Physiologists were able to perform their experiments in continuation of the tradition in laboratory practice, applying materials that came into general use in the last decades of the century. Of particular importance was the introduction of laboratory animals like guinea-pigs and rabbits, and somewhat later, mice and rats, which became the major subjects in their experiments to study the role of the ovaries and testes. The third group in the emerging field of sex hormones found it somewhat more difficult to gain access to research materials.[1] The pharmaceutical industry had no tradition or practice to lean on, so it had to make other arrangements. To obtain the material they needed for the production of testis and ovary preparations, pharmaceutical companies entered into contracts with local slaughterhouses to guarantee a steady supply of animal glands – organic matter that was not used for the production of food.

In this early period, the activities of the three groups involved in research on sex hormones did not interfere with one another. Every individual in these groups interested in the subject of sex hormones could enter the field and perform experiments without assistance or interference from other groups. In the early 1920s, however, the central focus in research shifted from the biological function to the chemical isolation and identification of sex hormones (Clarke 1985: 390). Unfortunately, the active substances scientists were seeking so desperately happened to occur only in small amounts in masses of inert matter (Parkes 1966). To obtain pure extracts, sex endocrinologists had to use tons of gonads. Gynecologists and laboratory scientists now had to devote much of their time to the search for large supplies of gonadal material. To understand how the three groups gradually became more and more dependent on one another, we can trace how they succeeded in meeting this new need.

Some scientists were very creative in finding a solution to the problem of obtaining large quantities of research materials. Alan Parkes, a physiologist at the National Institute for Medical Research in London, described how – thanks to the intervention of the British Museum – he was able to obtain ovaries from the southern blue whale. This enormous creature, weighing up to 70 tons, has correspondingly large ovaries: "a splendid opportunity of obtaining gonadal tissue in bulk." Unfortunately, a great deal of the precious material was lost because of bad preservation (Parkes 1985: 128). Similarly, Dutch scientists considered the use of whales' testes.

Because whales do not habitually swim near laboratories in the western world, this source was not a structural solution to the problem of scarcity. To gain access to the enormous quantities of required material, scientists had to create new infrastructural arrangements to secure a steady supply of organic matter. The previous arrangements in the laboratory and the clinic were no longer sufficient. To find access to research materials, laboratory scientists and gynecologists had to leave their laboratories and clinics. The most likely places where large quantities of ovaries and testes could be obtained were the slaughterhouses.[2]

This supply, however, was not equally accessible to all the groups involved in research on sex hormones. In this period the role of the pharmaceutical industry in the emerging field of sex endocrinology changed drastically. In the previous chapters, gynecologists and laboratory scientists were the major actors. Research on sex hormones was mainly located inside the laboratory and the clinic. In the making of sex hormones we see how the pharmaceutical industry became increasingly important in structuring the development of the study of sex hormones. We have seen how the pharmaceutical companies had already contracted with local slaughterhouses for the delivery of organic material, thus gaining control over an essential source of research materials. With these contracts, the pharmaceutical companies almost entirely blocked the access of others to this resource. Scientists often found pharmaceutical concerns to be their competitors in this quest. The American biochemist Edward Doisy described how he had to obtain permission from a pharmaceutical company to purchase ovaries, because this company had a contract with the local packing plant (Doisy 1972). To gain access to the supply of gonads present in slaughterhouses, gynecologists and laboratory scientists had to ally themselves with the pharmaceutical companies. Both in Germany and the United States, gynecologists and laboratory scientists created networks with pharmaceutical companies connected to slaughterhouses, thus guaranteeing a steady supply of gonadal material (Tausk 1978: 29–32).

DUTCH SEX ENDOCRINOLOGY

In The Netherlands, the infrastructural arrangements show a slightly different pattern that is very illustrative in clarifying how the networks between scientists and the pharmaceutical companies were built. Dutch scientists could not ally themselves with the pharmaceutical industry simply because no Dutch pharmaceutical company then existed. This situation forced scientists to opt for the strongest form of alliance they could create – namely, to take part in the founding of a pharmaceutical company.

The leading Dutch research group in the emerging field of endocrinology was the Pharmaco-Therapeutic Laboratory of the University of Amsterdam. This group consisted of physiologists, physicians and chemists, and was headed by Ernst Laqueur (Figure 4.1). Laqueur was born in Obernigk (Breslau) in 1880, and trained as a physician at the Universities of Breslau and Heidelberg. Besides his medical training he was educated in physical and organic chemistry and pharmacology. After several appointments at German and Belgian universities, he became professor of pharmacology at the University of Amsterdam in 1920 (Anonymous 1938). In memorials, Laqueur is usually described as an excellent manager, a scientist who did not shine so much in laboratory experiments but was a brilliant organizer of scientific labor (Tausk 1978: 12). This is obvious from the way in which he knew how to solve the problem of gaining access to research materials.

In 1923, Ernst Laqueur made contacts with Saal van Zwanenberg, the director of a Dutch slaughterhouse. At that time Zwanenberg – following a tradition that already existed in other countries – was looking for customers for the organic remains from his slaughterhouse. Among the waste products, mostly organs that could not be used for the production of food, were the glands of the slaughtered animals. This meeting marked the start of the founding of Organon. In June 1923, Ernst Laqueur signed a contract with Zwanenberg's Slaughterhouses and Fabrics Limited Company in which Laqueur was made scientific consultant for the preparation of medical organ products. Organon committed itself to processing the organic material from Zwanenberg's slaughterhouse. The Organon Limited Company was founded in July 1923, starting as a small laboratory inside the buildings of Zwanenberg's Slaughterhouse. The full name of this new company was: Organon Limited Company for the Manufacturing of Organ Preparations on a Scientific Basis. The very name of Organon was most probably suggested by Laqueur, having in mind the Greek word for organ. Laqueur became one of the three members of the board of directors, specifically in charge of the scientific and medical management of the company (Tausk 1978: 15, 17, 19).

In this manner, Ernst Laqueur solved the problem of acquiring research materials. Now the Amsterdam School was guaranteed a steady and reliable supply of all the organic material required for research, both on the pancreatic hormone (insulin) and on gonadal hormones. Through the 1920s and 1930s, Laqueur's laboratory maintained its close cooperation with Organon: the connection proved to be of great research value, not

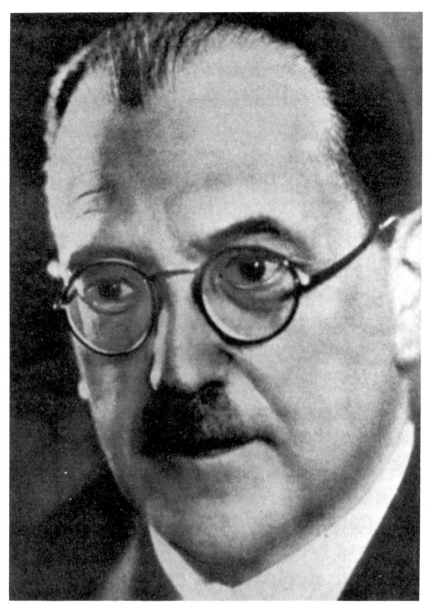

Figure 4.1 Professor Dr Ernst Laqueur
Source: Organon Archives

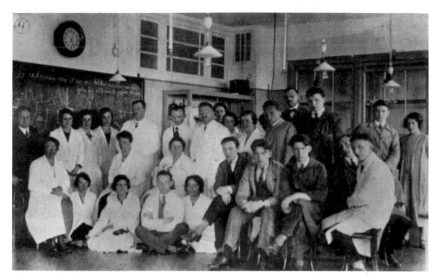

Figure 4.2 The staff of the Pharmaco-Therapeutic Laboratory at the University
of Amsterdam in 1926
Source: Organon Archives

only for the supply of gonads, but also when gonads were replaced by
urine as a source of pure hormones (Figure 4.2).

NETWORKS BETWEEN LABORATORY SCIENTISTS AND
PHARMACEUTICAL COMPANIES

The creation of networks between scientists and pharmaceutical companies was of central importance to research on sex hormones. The data
suggest that those scientists who had succeeded in making arrangements
with pharmaceutical industries formed the leading research groups in the
new study of sex hormones. All three of the research groups that first
isolated a pure female sex hormone worked in close cooperation with
pharmaceutical companies. The American biochemist Edward Doisy, who
reported the isolation of a crystalline estrogenic hormone to the Fifteenth
International Physiology Congress held in Boston in 1929, cooperated
with Parke, Davis, and Company. The work of the German biochemist
Adolf Butenandt, who reported the isolation of the same hormone two
months later, was supported by the Schering-Kalhbaum Company. Early
in the following year, Ernst Laqueur supported by Organon, also isolated
the hormone (Sneader 1985: 193–194).

Although the cooperation of laboratory scientists with pharmaceutical
companies had major advantages, relationships with pharmaceutical com-

panies could also be difficult, in particular in respect of the funding of research by grant agencies. In The Netherlands, the close connection between a private company like Organon and a university laboratory like the Pharmaco-Therapeutic Laboratory was often criticized, both inside and outside the scientific community. In 1931, the cooperation between Ernst Laqueur and Organon became a topic of debate in the City Council of Amsterdam, when Laqueur was called to account for the financial consequences of his connection with Organon. Laqueur had to convince the City Council that the municipal financial budget allocated to the Pharmaco-Therapeutic Laboratory in Amsterdam was not being (indirectly) spent on scientific equipment for Organon.[3] In this debate, Laqueur also described the role of Organon in supplying his laboratory with the required research materials:

> Large quantities of material are needed before substances can be obtained in a pure condition. The pharmaceutical laboratory does not have the means to purchase the required materials. Organon provides livers, urine and testes and whatever else might be needed for research. ... This cooperation is of importance both for the Pharmaco-Thera-peutic Laboratory and for Organon. If University Regulations were to prohibit professors from providing consultation, this would disadvan-tage the University, and the laboratory would not have much to show in terms of scientific results.[4]

Evaluating the developments in the 1920s, we can conclude that the quest for access to research materials had a significant impact on the research network and the strategic position of each group. During the 1920s, the relative independence of the previous decades was replaced by a strong interdependence of those involved in research on sex hormones. Labora-tory scientists and gynecologists had become dependent on the pharma-ceutical companies for the supply of research materials. The pharmaceutical companies gained the strategic position of controlling the supply of these materials. However, the pharmaceutical companies in turn, as well as the gynecologists, had to rely on the laboratory scientists. As we saw in Chapter 3, the laboratory scientists had achieved the strategic position of possessing biological assay techniques to guarantee the quality of commercial hormone products. Thus, in addition to the supply of research materials, the availibility of techniques also had an impact on the inter-relationships between the groups, strengthening the network created around the research materials. In the course of the 1920s, the character of the relationships between the groups thus shifted from one of critical partners sharing a common interest to one in which the groups were heavily dependent on one another to gain access to research materials.

THE QUEST FOR OVARIES AND FEMALE URINE

Although the problem of gaining access to research materials had been solved, scientists continued searching for new sources. The main reason for this was the enormous expense of gonadal material.[5] Scientists working on female sex hormones were eager to find sources less expensive than cows' ovaries. Horse ovaries happened to be less expensive than cows' ovaries, but horse ovaries were not easily available because few horses were slaughtered at that time. Another possible source was the human placenta. Owing to the expense and scarcity of ovaries, many investigators turned their attention to this more abundant and relatively inexpensive source (Doisy 1939: 848). However, this source was not a good substitute for cows' ovaries because placental extracts could not be purified to the same extent as ovarian extracts.

But the quest for new sources would soon take a happy turn. In 1926, two German scientists happened to find the long-sought-for source: human urine (Corner 1965: 15). S. Ascheim, a gynecologist at the Gyneco-Pathological Laboratory of the City Hospital in Berlin, was involved in developing diagnostic tests for disorders in menstruation and fertility (Zondek and Finkelstein 1966: 6). Gynecologists analyzed blood, and later urine, to detect differences in hormonal content between healthy women and their patients.[6] Together with his colleague Bernhard Zondek, Ascheim also analyzed urine from their pregnant patients. This last endeavor would turn out to be the moment that many colleagues had eagerly awaited. Urine from pregnant women – even in the raw state – happened to be far more active than the best ovarian extracts so far obtained.[7] Bernhard Zondek acknowledged the relevance of their achievement for his colleagues outside gynecology. Through his connections with the Dutch pharmaceutical company Organon, Zondek promoted this new source.[8]

The discovery of Ascheim and Zondek had a significant impact on the relationship between the three groups involved in research on female sex hormones. In this period, the gynecologists regained a somewhat stronger position in the emerging field of sex endocrinology. To gain access to the new source of urine, the actors had to rely on the gynecologists: scientists could obtain the urine of pregnant women only from gynecological clinics. This became a new source of inexpensive and easily available material for research on female sex hormones,[9] and signaled the end of the period in which research was constrained by the scarcity of research materials. Urine proved to be an ideal source. As a liquid, it could be extracted with ease; owing to its composition there were only small amounts of inert products in the extract; and what was even more important, the supply of urine was both abundant and inexpensive.

In addition, the position of the laboratory scientists changed radically during this period. With the introduction of urine, chemical analytical methods became more important: the new discipline of biochemistry consequently became increasingly involved in research on sex hormones. The biochemists had mastered one technique that gynecologists and their colleagues in the laboratory did not possess – the technique of making invisible female and male substances visible. Following the discovery of Ascheim and Zondek, chemists devoted their energies to the isolation of female sex hormones from the urine of pregnant women. The new source stimulated chemical work, and turned out to be one of the major factors contributing to the isolation and chemical identification of female sex hormones (Doisy 1939: 851). Within less than three years from Ascheim and Zondek's 1926 publication, European and American research groups reported the isolation and identification of female sex hormone from the urine of pregnant women.

The use of urine as a research material reinforced the relationship between scientists and the pharmaceutical industry. Although the use of urine solved many problems, individual scientists still had to spend quite some time in collecting the material they needed.[10] Those scientists working in close cooperation with pharmaceutical industries could profit once more from this relationship. In some cases the pharmaceutical company undertook both the collection and the processing of pregnant women's urine.[11] Scientists could simply obtain the extracted hormones from the companies.

In this period, laboratory scientists were strengthening their position. With the introduction of urine and the application of chemical methods, research gradually shifted from the gynecologists to the laboratory scientists. The individual gynecologist of the earlier days, experimenting on a small scale with extracts prepared from ovaries obtained from the clinic, was replaced by laboratory scientists working with enormous quantities of research material provided by the pharmaceutical companies.

In the years to come, gynecologists also lost their strategic position as suppliers. In 1930, Zondek suggested that the urine of pregnant mares was superior to human urine as a source of female sex hormones. Now scientists were no longer dependent on the gynecological clinic to obtain the material they needed. This did not in itself greatly affect the direction of research, because the estrogenic hormone had already been isolated from the urine of pregnant women. The "second" female sex hormone, progesterone, was isolated in 1934 from animal ovaries (Parkes 1966: 23). However, the urine of pregnant mares turned out to be of great importance for the commercial production of female sex hormones by pharmaceutical companies, for it was even less expensive than human urine (Figure 4.3). For the second time, Organon followed Zondek's advice (Tausk 1978: 32). In the years to follow, Organon processed millions of liters of mares' urine (an operation that could not remain unnoticed by the people living near the factory!). To collect this urine, Organon organized special campaigns among horse owners.[12] One can imagine that farmers (and even the Ministry of Agriculture) were most surprised to discover that they could sell the liquid waste products from their mares for prices equal to those of cows' milk (Tausk 1978: 119).

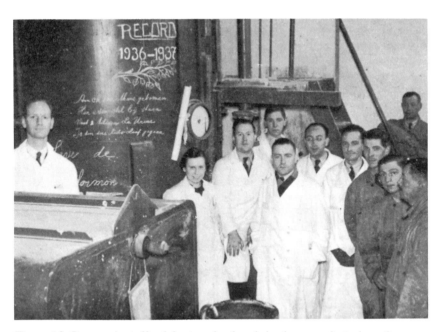

Figure 4.3 Organon's staff celebrate a landmark in the manufacturing of *Menformon* (female sex hormone) in the 1936–1937 working season: the use of the millionth liter of mares' urine
Source: Organon Archives

Clearly, the introduction of urine had an impact on the position of the three groups. In the late 1920s and the early 1930s, research on female sex hormones definitely shifted from the clinic to the laboratory. Although gynecologists had temporarily strengthened their position as suppliers of female urine, they totally lost their position in research on sex hormones. The laboratory scientists and the pharmaceutical companies, however, strengthened their positions in the network. Thus, of the three groups previously involved in research on female sex hormones, only two retained their position: the pharmaceutical companies and the laboratory scientists. Moreover, inside the laboratory a shift in positions had also taken place: after the late 1920s, biochemists became increasingly involved in the subject of sex hormones, and partly took over the subject from the physiologists who had done the pioneer work in the laboratory (Corner 1965: 4, 15).[13]

THE QUEST FOR TESTES AND MALE URINE

The success story of access to new sources for female sex hormones cannot be told about male sex hormones. Research on male sex hormones was far more constrained by the limited availability of organic material than was research on female sex hormones. In the early years, female gonads had been relatively easy for gynecologists to obtain because human ovaries were regularly removed in the clinic (Zondek and Finkelstein 1966: 6). However, no comparable clinical practice, in which healthy or affected testes were removed, existed for the male body (T. Laqueur 1990: 176). Consequently, human testes were very difficult to obtain. Scientists even awaited executions in prisons to gather these materials (Hamilton 1986). This difficulty led to the search for other sources of male hormones. After the isolation of female sex hormones from the urine of pregnant women in 1929, it was not surprising that laboratory scientists began to examine human urine for male sex hormones (Koch 1939).

Remarkably, the availability of urine as a source to obtain male sex hormones did not have the same impact on research as it had had on research on female sex hormones. Male urine was a suitable source in theory, but not in practice, simply because there was no institutional context for its collection, as there was for female urine. Men's clinics specializing in the study of the male reproductive system did not exist in the 1920s. The collection of urine from male patients in normal hospitals could not solve the problem, because the content of male sex hormones in the urine of sick males turned out to be much lower than in the urine of healthy men (J. Freud 1930). Nor was animal urine a solution, because it contained very little male hormone. Human urine appeared to be unique with respect to male hormonal content (Gustavson 1939). Thus scientists remained totally dependent on human male urine.

How did scientists eventually gain access to male urine? To collect it, scientists had to look for institutions other than the clinic – places where men regularly gathered, like big factories or other male occupational spheres. In 1931, the German chemist Adolf Butenandt collected 25,000 liters of men's urine in the police barracks in Berlin, from which he isolated 50 mg of a crystalline substance to which he subsequently gave the name "androsterone" in the belief that it was the essential male hormone (Parkes 1966: 25). However, this supply of male urine was quite problematic. Scientists had to rely on the delivery of male urine from institutions in which the collection of urine was not a common practice. Both German and Dutch scientists described how difficult it was to gain access to male urine in these institutions. Butenandt's colleague Koch described how it took Butenandt two years before he could obtain enough material to revise the formulae and potency of the male sex hormone he had isolated in 1931. (Koch 1936) Laqueur, in his function as a member of the board of Organon, had to take great pains to obtain permission from the Ministry of Defence and the directors of prisons to collect male urine in military barracks and penitentiaries. In 1930, Laqueur addressed the Ministry of Defence, formulating his request as follows:

> In order to produce male sex hormone preparations, it is absolutely necessary to have access to a large quantity of raw material, in this case a large amount of urine from not too elderly men. Although this material is abundant in rather huge quantities and has the additional advantage of being valueless, it is very difficult to collect.... The production of female sex hormones only succeeded thanks to the cooperation of directors of women's clinics and midwife schools. In concluding, I want to emphasize the scientific and therapeutic interests that are at stake and that legitimize your cooperation in order to obtain the required raw material from the barracks.[14]

Organon first obtained male urine from its German subsidiary in Berlin, Degewop; later Organon obtained the urine from Dutch factories, military barracks and penitentiaries.[15] The supply of male urine remained, however, problematic. Laqueur again, in 1933:

> Hombreol is very expensive, because large quantities of raw material are required for the production of this hormone. The collection and transport of the large quantities of male urine is very difficult and expensive.

> (Capellen 1936)

Thus, scientists had once again to rely on the pharmaceutical companies for their supply. In Germany, the collection and processing of the urine was carried out by the pharmaceutical company Schering AG (Tausk 1978: 56). Dutch scientists could profit once more from their close cooperation with Organon, which provided them with the large quantities of urine required for research on male sex hormones.

It was only when male sex hormones could be made synthetically, and organic materials were no longer needed, that an increase took place in research on male sex hormones. The chemical characterization of male sex hormones, and their synthesis in 1936, made possible a burst of biochemical and biological work (Parkes 1966: 25; Tschopp 1935). At last scientists could easily gain access to male sex hormones. The pharmaceutical companies could provide them with any quantity of synthetic male sex hormones they needed. Research was stimulated by the distribution of a wide range of male sex hormones by the pharmaceutical companies (Parkes 1966: 25).[16] The number of research publications on male sex hormones that appeared in the 1920s and 1930s indicates the impact of this synthetic supply.[17]

The chemical identification of sex hormones also provided scientists with the means to synthesize modified sex hormones. This specific episode in the history of male sex hormones illustrates nicely that sex hormones are not entities that only had to be "discovered" in nature (i.e. biological material), but that sex hormones were objects constructed in the laboratory as materializations of particular ideas about what sex hormones should look like. With the influx of biochemists into the field of sex hormones, the purification of these substances evolved into one of the major aims of research in the 1930s. In this process of purification, scientists were, however, confronted with specific problems. Purified preparations of testes and male urine did not produce the responses expected from male sex hormone. In 1937, Laqueur's research group described these problems:

> It is evident now that these preparations produce only a very moderate growth of the sexual organs in castrated infantile rats and mice, compared to what we reasonably would have expected. We succeeded, however, in strengthening the activity of male sex hormones ... by means of the addition of estrone [at that time still known as the female sex hormone *par excellence*!]. A complete substitution for the testes remained, however, an unapproachable ideal. ... It cannot be denied that the esterification of male hormone preparations has led to substances which almost reach our ideal of a "male hormone": the complete restitution of the castrate is no longer impossible, at least in animal experiments.
>
> (Jongh 1937: 43)

Because the purified hormone preparations of organic material did not have the quality scientists expected, chemists constructed the male sex hormone by the esterification of testes preparations. Thus, only by chemical modification could scientists materialize the "ideal male sex hormone". In 1934, Marius Tausk, the medical director of Organon, evaluated this development in the field of sex hormones:

> The time has passed in which hormones were mythical substances. More and more we become informed about the chemical structure of these important elements of the organism, and science not only introduces the synthetic production of hormones, but also constructs transformations in the molecule, in order to improve the activity of the natural substances. Evidently, man attempts to be wiser than nature itself.
>
> (Tausk 1934a: 46)

Summarizing the quest for male sex hormones, we can conclude that in this case (even more than for female sex hormones), laboratory scientists had to rely on the pharmaceutical companies to provide them with the required material. In contrast with female sex hormones, the study of male sex hormones was dominated from the beginning by two groups – the laboratory scientists and the pharmaceutical companies. The gynecologists were more interested in the role of the ovaries in female disorders and focused only on the study of female sex hormones.

RESEARCH MATERIALS AS CARRIERS OF KNOWLEDGE CLAIMS

What was the impact of the making of sex hormones on the conceptualization of sex differences? To answer this question I have to highlight another function of research materials. Not only did the availability of research materials have an impact on the interrelationship between the groups involved in research on sex hormones, but also research materials functioned as carriers in the transmission, and consequently the selection of knowledge claims. To understand the role of research materials in the development of research, we can trace the movement of research materials from one group to another.

In the period of the introduction of the concept of sex hormones, the three groups involved in research on sex hormones focussed on different research questions. The gynecologists were particularly interested in the role of female sex hormones in female disorders associated with the ovaries, and in processes of reproduction in the female body. Gynecologists tentatively began to wonder if and how the internal secretions of the ovaries might control ovulation, menstruation and pregnancy. The pharmaceutical companies followed up these claims by producing ovarian preparations for therapeutic purposes. The laboratory scientists shared a broader interest. Besides issues of reproduction, laboratory scientists were particularly interested in the role of both female and male sex hormones in the growth and development of the body in general, and more specifically in the process of sexual differentiation – the development and maintenance of both the sexual organs and the secondary sexual characteristics.

In the early period, when the three groups still worked independently from one another, all claims were investigated with equal attention. This situation changed drastically from the moment the groups had to rely on each other for the supply of research materials. With the transfer of research materials from one group to another, knowledge claims specific to the group in control of the research materials were also transferred. In this process a selection of knowledge claims took place: some claims became stronger, others weaker.

The first time this happened was in the period when scientists were using human female gonads in their research. Only the gynecologists could easily gain access to this type of research material. To translate their claims from animals to human organisms, all groups had to rely on the gynecological clinic, as the only place where human gonads could be obtained. Here we see the first selection of claims. The claims attached to the male gonads could not be transferred from animals to humans because a medical practice for the provision of human testes did not exist. In this way, the knowledge claims that gynecologists attached to female sex hormones became stronger than the claims of the other groups. Thus, claims concerning the role of female sex hormones in female disorders and female reproduction gained more momentum than claims concerning sexual differentiation and male reproductive functions.

This initial selection of claims was further reinforced in the period when scientists began to use human urine. As we have seen, human urine as a source of research materials stimulated research on female sex hormones enormously, because female urine could easily be obtained and processed. Because the gynecologists could gain access to the urine of women more easily than the other groups, the process of selection of claims was further strengthened in the direction of their own interests. With the transfer of the urine of their female patients from the gynecological clinic to the laboratory and the pharmaceutical companies, the claims concerning women's diseases and reproduction were also transferred. Particularly during the period when urine was becoming established as a source of research materials, claims about the interrelationships between female sex hormones, women's diseases and reproduction became stronger: gradually, they became the major focus on the research agenda of the three groups.

Because both methods and research materials were well developed and easily available, more and more scientists became involved in research on female sex hormones. Through the 1920s and 1930s, the number of publications on female sex hormones increased steadily, and far outnumbered those on male sex hormones.[18] In the urinary period, both the laboratory scientists and the pharmaceutical companies became definitely committed to the specific interests of the gynecologists in female sex hormones. Since the 1920s, all three groups have shared a mutual interest in female sex hormones as a field that has gradually developed into big science and big business.

Summarizing the role of research materials in the development of sex endocrinology, we can conclude that in the selection process of knowledge claims that resulted from the transfer of research materials, women and reproduction became the central focus of research. In the triangle gynecology-laboratory-pharmaceutical industry, the male gradually disappeared from the forefront as an object of research. Although most actors were male, the object of research was almost entirely female. Knowledge claims linking men with reproduction could not be stabilized because there did not exist an institutional context for the study of the process of reproduction in men. Although the need for the establishment of a separate and distinct specialty for the study of the male reproductive system was suggested as early as 1891, not until the late 1960s was andrology institutionalized as a medical specialty.[19] These differences in the institutionalization of the life sciences exerted an all-pervasive impact on the development of reproductive research. Consequently, the development of knowledge about male reproduction was long delayed.[20]

CONCLUSIONS

This focus on the material conditions for hormone research highlights a feature that is of major importance in the development of science. Scientists do not construct facts and artefacts isolated from their social context. In order to make sex hormones, scientists had to create networks with other social groups outside the laboratory. The construction of sex hormones took place in networks formed between three groups: the laboratory, the clinic and the pharmaceutical industry. These networks were of vital importance in the study of sex hormones. Had laboratory scientists not succeeded in capturing the interests of the pharmaceutical industry, research on sex hormones would have stayed inside the walls of the laboratory.

Research materials played a crucial role in the building of these networks. This reconstruction illustrates how research materials became the pivot on which the relationships among the different groups involved in the making of sex hormones hinged. By tracing how scientists gained access to research materials, it became obvious how the different groups, at first operating independently, gradually became enmeshed in a network of dependences and alliances. The nature of their relationship changed from one of independence to one of mutual dependence. Research materials functioned as an organizing medium, bringing the groups together and shaping the relationships between them. Research materials were thus instrumental in linking the practices of the laboratory to their social context: the clinic and the pharmaceutical industry.

This reconstruction also illustrates how the scientific endeavor produces not only theoretical claims. Through a close cooperation with the pharmaceutical companies, laboratory scientists transformed the theoretical concept of sex hormones into material realities: chemical products that could circulate outside the walls of the laboratories. In this respect, there remains one major question to be answered: what happened when sex hormones left the laboratory? In the next chapter we follow the laboratory scientists, the pharmaceutical companies and the medical profession in the next phase of the creation of sex hormones: the transformation of sex hormones into specific drugs.

5 The marketing of sex hormones

You don't have to be a very keen observer to notice that today hormones are everywhere: not only in our language but also in hospitals, chemists' shops, even in women's dressing-cases. The introduction of the hormonal model of the body has been very successful, particularly for women. Women all over the world take hormonal pills to control their fertility, for menstrual or menopausal problems, or as abortifacients. The hormones estrogen and progesterone have become so popular that they have developed into the most widely used drugs in the history of medicine (Wolffers *et al.* 1989).

How can we understand this success story? What intrigues me most is that it is the female body that became increasingly subjected to hormonal treatment. What about men and hormones? Maybe we might be inclined to think of a male conspiracy: women take the pills, while men cash the bills. We might consider the enormous profits of pharmaceutical firms. To be honest, I am not very much attracted to these types of explanations, particularly because they do not give us any insight in how the medicalization of women's bodies takes place. Recently, feminist scholars have suggested that feminist inquiry should go "beyond the inadequate but often terminal analysis that men are the problem" (Clarke 1990a: 10; Haraway 1988: 575). Interpretations of the successes of science and technology, whether they are framed in terms of the interests of men or pharmaceutical firms, suffer from the same problem: they consider interests as a given, a reality that does not need any further explanation.[1] However, if we adopt the view that the natural world is not objectively given, it seems inconsistent to make an exception for the social world. I am more in favor of an approach that enables us to conceptualize both worlds as social constructions that are continuously shaped and transformed by human actions. Interests, just as facts, are not objectively given but collectively created.

What I would like to know is how interests are shaped together with the technology-in-the-making, in this case the making of hormones into drugs. I chose to focus on clinical trials as a specific site where the shaping of technologies and interests takes place. A crucial aspect of the process of drug development is that one specific working pattern is selected from a large number of possibilities. This selection process takes place in specific test procedures (clinical trials) in which the drug profile – as it were, the "nature" of the drug – is defined (Vos 1989: 278). The question that emerges now is how and when this testing takes place. Social studies of medical technologies provide two strands of explanation for how we can understand the development of medical technologies such as drugs. The sequential or linear model of technology development assumes that technologies are thoroughly tested before being adopted. This model suggests that the testing procedure in which the final drug profile is selected takes place prior to the marketing of drugs. More recent studies of the development of medical technologies suggest, however, that technologies are usually adopted before they have been thoroughly tested. This literature suggests that the diffusion of new drugs occurs together with research and testing (Bell 1986: 5).

The adoption of this model of technology development enables us to understand technologies and interests as products of mutual alliances and dependencies among the groups involved in the testing and marketing of medical technologies. In this view hormonal drugs are neither ready-made laboratory products that are subsequently marketed to their audiences, nor are they compounds simply discovered in nature. The specific "nature" of the drug and the interests that become embodied in it are shaped in the networks of the different groups that called hormonal drugs into existence. I describe how the making of hormonal drugs took place in the triangle of the laboratory, the pharmaceutical industry and the clinic, with clinical trials and advertising strategies as major marketing devices. To understand how these groups transformed sex hormones into specialized drugs, I shall focus once again on The Netherlands. This chapter begins with a brief description of the position of the Dutch pharmaceutical company Organon. Next I analyze in detail the promotion of sex hormones by Organon and Laqueur, focusing on the specific patterns of medical therapeutics for women and men that emerged from this joint venture.

ORGANON: A SCIENCE-BASED COMPANY

Nowadays, Organon is one of the leading pharmaceutical firms in the market of hormonal drugs (Tausk 1978: 35; Wolffers *et al.* 1989: 32). This position dates from the 1920s, when the Dutch company gained a strong position in the industrial market as a major producer of female sex hormones, a position it held till the Second World War. Organon's first product appeared on the market in 1923. This was not a sex hormone, but the pancreatic hormone, insulin. Insulin was considered a "respectable" drug for a well-defined disease (diabetes). With this new drug

Organon established its position as a pharmaceutical company in The Netherlands.

Since its foundation in 1923, Organon has presented itself as a science-based company, explicitly expressed in its corporate slogan: "Manufacturer of Organ Preparations on a Scientific Basis" (Figure 5.1).

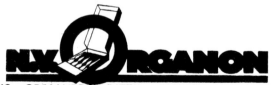

TOT BEREIDING van ORGAANPREPARATEN op WETENSCHAPPELIJKEN GRONDSLAG

TELEFOON INTERC. 1 EN 3
TELEGRAMADRES:
ORGANON OSS

POSTREKENING NR. 110914
BANKIER AMSTERDAMSCHE
BANK · NIJMEGEN

CODES: RUDOLF MOSSE
BENTLEY, ABC VI.

Am@S8rdam 23 Mei 1929
(HOLLAND)

N.V.Organon
O.S.S

REF.:

Figure 5.1
Organon's letterhead: Organon Limited Company for the Manufacturing of Organ Preparations on a Scientific Basis.
Source: Organon Archives

The image of a scientific company was chosen as a general strategy in approaching clinicians and general practitioners.[2] By emphasizing its scientific character, Organon tried to clear the clouds of illegitimacy and quackery hanging over previous organ preparations, and sought to convince the medical profession of the superior quality of its products. Since the 1890s organotherapy had become rather popular and gave rise to a flourishing trade in organ extracts from virtually all tissues. Notwithstanding its popularity, the medical application of extracts of animal organs, however, remained rather controversial. The clinical promise that animal extracts would provide drugs for the treatment of a wide variety of diseases ascribed to malfunctions of the corresponding organ, was not fulfilled as readily as scientists had expected. In the early years of organotherapy only thyroid and adrenal extracts were considered to be of therapeutic value. During the following decades, organotherapy became increasingly associated with "quackery." The evaluation of gonadal extracts was even more controversial because of Brown-Séquard's claims about rejuvenation and sexuality (Borell 1985). The controversy about organotherapy also had major advantages. The debate about the therapeutic value of organ extracts brought this new type of drug into the limelight. Subsequently, the study of organ extracts and their therapeutic promise was known throughout the world at the turn of the century (Clarke 1989).

We saw before how criticism of the therapeutic value of organ preparations was part of the broader debate about the quality of all types of drugs, that was initiated by the medical profession in their striving for a "scientific" medicine at the turn of the century (Clarke 1989). In the 1920s, Dutch general practitioners founded the Society against Quackery (de Vereniging tegen Kwakzalverij) to protest against the "growing anarchy in drugs" (Pinkhof 1927a; 1927b). Following the debate on quackery, drug regulation gradually became institutionalized. The Netherlands was among the first countries to establish a special institute for the control of drugs. In 1920, the Dutch authorities founded the Government Institute for Pharmaco-therapeutic Research (not to be confused with Laqueur's laboratory) for the control and inspection of the quality of commercial pharmaceutical products. The task of this institute was "to investigate the composition, purity, and pharmacological activity of drugs, disinfectants, and food, which are used in the cure of diseases."[3] Following these drug regulations, pharmaceutical companies had to labor under more rigid constraints.

The institutionalization of drug control in The Netherlands had a major impact on Organon's policy with respect to the promotion of its products. In order to avoid association with quackery, Organon adopted the strategy of addressing the medical profession and not the public. As the medical profession became increasingly science-oriented, so Organon emphasized the scientific character of its products.[4] Hormone preparations were promoted as scientific medicines, not as folk medicines. The close cooperation of Organon with Laqueur's laboratory strengthened the scientific image of Organon.

To interest general practitioners and clinicians in the new area of hormone therapy and to convince them of its scientific character, Organon founded a specific journal, entitled *Het Hormoon* (*The Hormone*). This journal was founded in 1931 by Organon's medical director, Marius Tausk, who edited the journal for almost twenty years; in the early years he also wrote most of the articles (published unsigned). The aim of *Het Hormoon* was "to provide a summary of published literature and – as we hope – a not too dry reproduction from this. This reproduction will take place objectively and according to scientific points of view." (Tausk 1978: 102). Initially restricted to The Netherlands, the journal was soon published in French, German, English, Czech, Polish and Italian, and distributed gratis in more than ten different countries all over Europe (Tausk 1935: 1). This journal played a major role in informing the medical profession about hormones as drugs, especially since drug information, other than that supplied by companies, was not abundant in those years. In the 1920s, the pharmaceutical industry was one of the major suppliers on information of drugs, in Europe as well as in the United States. In the USA physicians relied heavily on pharmaceutical firms to provide the most recent information about new products. Sometimes the medical journals published

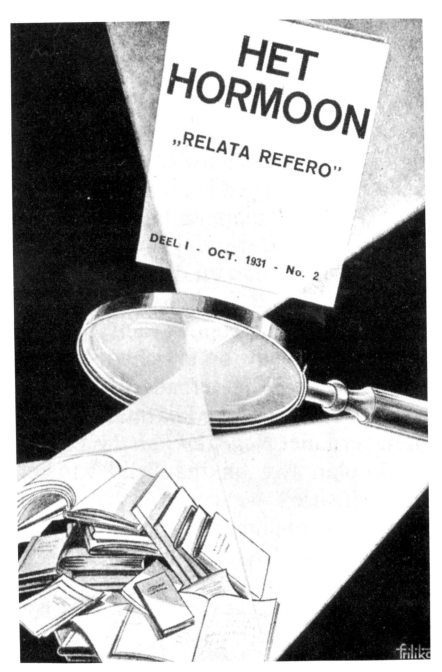

Figure 5.2   The first cover of Organon's journal *Het Hormoon (The Hormone)*.
Source: Organon Archives

independent results of clinical tests, but this was not always the case. Moreover, the reports in medical journals were often far less complete than the information provided by pharmaceutical companies (Liebenau 1987: 129). *Het Hormoon* thus functioned as a major device to control the flow of information about this new class of drugs to the medical profession (Figure 5.2).

The strategy of Organon to present itself as a science-based industry was not just designed to establish a scientific veneer. Cooperation with university scientists provided Organon with all the means required to develop into a major science-based industry. We have seen how the cooperation with laboratory scientists provided the pharmaceutical company with the required biological assay techniques to manufacture hormonal preparations which, in contrast to previous products made by other companies, could meet the scientific standards of quality. From the start, Organon had a small laboratory, housing equipment transferred from Laqueur's laboratory. Research on sex hormones took place both at Organon's laboratory in Oss and at Laqueur's laboratory in Amsterdam. In this period, there was as yet no strong division between manufacturing and research, because all manufacturing procedures were practically new, and thus required much basic research (Tausk 1978: 52). Organon's laboratory staff was trained at Laqueur's laboratory. Moreover, the hormone preparations produced by Organon were controlled for quality in the laboratory in Amsterdam and were put on the market only with the permission of Laqueur. Ernst Laqueur had the right of veto over hormone preparations that were not passed by his laboratory (Tausk 1978: 16). Laqueur thus provided Organon with access to procedures for testing, standardizing and synthesizing its products, which enabled the young firm to establish its position in the industrial market of hormones.

The alliance with Organon also brought important benefits to Laqueur. In addition to delivering research materials, Organon paid well for his expertise, thus enabling Laqueur to expand his laboratory staff. Most importantly, Organon provided Laqueur with a window to the outside world, from which he could mass-produce and subsequently transfer sex hormones from the laboratory to the market. In the next sections, we shall follow Organon and Laqueur in their joint venture to market female and male sex hormones as new types of drugs in the 1920s and 1930s.

THE PROMOTION OF FEMALE SEX HORMONES

Early expectations and clinical trials

The marketing of female sex hormones was characterized by an atmosphere of high expectations. Ernst Laqueur described the joint venture of his laboratory and Organon as "the pursuit of the Goddess of Fortune"

(E. Laqueur *et al.* 1927a). What kind of goddess were scientists seeking? What type of medicine did they expect to find?

In 1925, Laqueur described the hormone they so eagerly sought for as "the hormone of the female menstruation cycle" (Organon Archive 8 November 1925). This expectation is also reflected in the name that Laqueur chose for Organon's first standardized female sex hormone preparation: *Menformon*, derived from the Latin words *mensis* (month) and *formare* (to make), meaning to make the menstruation.[5]

In the United States the medical profession raised similar expectations. Robert Frank described these in *The Female Sex Hormone* (published in 1929):

> Since 1923 the subject of female sex hormones has attracted innumerable workers who are elbowing and jostling each other and jockeying for position in the neck and neck race to isolate and synthesize the much desired and long sought for hormone, which is bound to relieve many of the ills from which women suffer.
>
> (Frank 1929: Introduction)

In his promotion of female sex hormones Laqueur followed the dualistic model, according to which sex hormones were conceptualized as sexually specific in origin and function, and he directed female sex hormone therapy strictly toward women. The expectation of manufacturing a medicine for the treatment of all diseases generally described as "women's diseases" indicated a very promising market, since this therapy could be extended to all women. It is thus not surprising that Marius Tausk described the chemical isolation and identification of the female sex hormone as "finding gold in the urine of pregnant mares," one of the sources from which scientists derived hormonal preparations (Tausk 1978: 116).

Early expectations of the therapeutic value of female sex hormones were inextricably enmeshed with cultural ideals about femininity. In Germany, female sex hormones (trade name *Ovowop*) were advertised with the slogan: "Women's declining, will return with Ovowop" (Tausk 1978: 57). This dream of finding a medical therapy to induce eternal femininity is also reflected in the trade name *Neogynon*, suggested by Laqueur "because female sex hormones stimulate femininity and beauty" (Organon Archive 29 September 1925).

How did Organon put its first female sex hormone preparation on the market? And which market was it? Although expectations were high, the therapeutic value of female sex hormones was still largely unexplored. To whom did Organon expect to sell this new type of drug, one still not connected to any clearly defined illness? Before the actual decision was made, Laqueur tested the hormone preparation for toxicity among what he described as "five healthy persons, two women and three men," consisting of Laqueur himself and four of his colleagues at the Pharmaco-

Therapeutic Laboratory in Amsterdam, which convinced him of its safety (Organon Archive 11 November 1925). In those days, the testing of hormone preparations by the scientists themselves as guinea-pigs was a generally accepted practice. Although Laqueur was convinced of its safety (obviously, because his colleagues did not complain of any negative effects), Ina Uyldert, a biologist who worked in Laqueur's laboratory after 1933, later described how she had been quite ill after the administration of rather large quantities of female sex hormones.[6] In January 1925, Organon decided to put its first female sex hormone preparation on the market, under the trade name *Ovarnon*, and began an advertising campaign (Organon Archive 1 January 1925). Organon and Laqueur discussed whether or not the campaign should be preceded by clinical trials to investigate the therapeutic activity of the drug. However, they decided that it was not necessary to wait for clinical results, and in February 1925, the first pamphlet was mailed to Dutch general practitioners (Organon Archive 7 February 1925).

The decision to start advertising before the results of clininal trials were known, and consequently having only vague ideas about the clinical activity of female sex hormones, can be understood in the context of the sharp competition among pharmaceutical companies eager to gain the leading position on the world market for this new drug, a competition mentioned already by Robert Frank.[7] The decision not to perform clinical trials accelerated the process of marketing considerably. Laqueur requested a patent for Organon as the sole producer of female sex hormones in September 1925.[8]

The advertising campaign to Dutch general practitioners did not solve the problem that Organon was promoting a drug of which the therapeutic value was largely unknown. The only strategy for gaining information about the therapeutic utility of female sex hormones was through the organization of clinical trials. In December 1925 Laqueur wrote to Organon:

> We can only learn by experience whether female sex hormone therapy will be of any clinical value. . . . Theoretically one cannot make the slightest prediction whether it will have any useful effects. In the end this will have to appear in practice.
>
> (Organon Archive 12 December 1925)

At this point, Organon and Laqueur were totally dependent on the willingness and cooperation of the medical profession. Which branch of the medical profession would be helpful in solving the question of the therapeutic value of female sex hormones? Organon decided to take the question to gynecological clinics. Gynecologists were already acquainted with the study of the ovaries, and some were actively involved in the study of female sex hormones. The gynecological clinic provided an institutional context in which Organon could organize clinical trials.

The first clinical trials were organized on a small scale. In January 1926 Laqueur approached the director of the gynecological clinic in Breslau, Germany (Organon Archive 5 January 1926). Born in Obernigk (Breslau) and trained as a physician at the University of Breslau, Laqueur was more acquainted with German clinicians than with their Dutch counterparts (Anonymous 1938). At the same time, Organon extended its advertising campaign to Germany. Laqueur also recommended *Ovarnon* to other gynecological clinics in Berlin (Organon Archive 8 November 1925). But the fact that the early clinical trials took place in Germany and not in The Netherlands was not only due to Laqueur's background. In a lecture to his colleagues in the Genootschap ter Bevordering van Natuur-, Genees- en Heelkunde (Society for the Promotion of Science, Medicine and Surgery) in 1926, Laqueur complained that interest in clinical trials in The Netherlands was much smaller than abroad. In this address, Laqueur also requested the cooperation of clinicians:

> Although therapeutic experiences are rather poor, it seems to us that it is now the task of the clinician to investigate the therapeutic effects of these preparations, which exert a specific biological activity in an area in which the clinician would like to exercise his influence.
>
> (E. Laqueur *et al.* 1927a: 2087–2,088)[9]

What kinds of medical indications were chosen for treatment with *Ovarnon*? Laqueur advised the German gynecological clinics to test *Ovarnon* first in female patients with menstrual disorders, in particular in cases in which menstruation was totally absent (amenorrhea).

In 1927 Laqueur extended the network to gynecological clinics in The Netherlands. One year after the initiation of clinical trials in Germany, Laqueur approached gynecologists from the Women's Clinics of the Universities of Amsterdam and Utrecht who, obviously inspired by Laqueur's lecture in 1926, were "very delighted and willing to cooperate in clinical trials" (Organon Archive 12 March 1927). Dutch gynecologists wondered whether female sex hormones "exerted a positive influence on the major female function: the cyclic changes in the genital apparatus with menstruation as a visible symptom" (Dongen 1929).

The organization of clinical trials in gynecological clinics was very much intertwined with the strategy of Organon to obtain the raw materials needed to manufacture hormone preparations. In this period, female urine had become the main source of raw materials for female sex hormones. Organon and Laqueur tried to gain the cooperation of Dutch gynecological clinics to deliver urine (and placentae) from their female patients. In exchange, Organon promised to distribute *Ovarnon* free of charge, for the purpose of arranging clinical trials. This was unusual: in earlier trials with other hormones (like insulin), the hormone preparations had been made available at manufacturing cost (Organon Archive 26 September 1927). In negotiations with clinics, Laqueur persuaded directors by emphasizing the benefits that gynecologists could reap by cooperating with Organon: "Clinics that cooperate will receive better hormone preparations for clinical trials than the preparations that are already on the market" (Organon Archive 26 September 1927).

Thus Organon gained twice from the cooperation with gynecological clinics: the network provided the institutional context for clinical trials as well as for the collection of raw materials.[10] In 1927, both Laqueur and Marius Tausk paid regular visits to gynecological clinics in Germany and The Netherlands in order to discuss the clinical trials and to make arrangements for the delivery of urine and placentae (Organon Archive 26 September and 7 October 1927). The gynecologists in turn could profit from the network with the pharmaceutical industry because Organon provided them with female sex hormone preparations free of charge. Moreover, the results of clinical trials were often published in Dutch journals (*Nederlands Tijdschrift voor Geneeskunde* and *Het Hormoon*), mostly under the name of the gynecologist, thus strengthening the image of gynecology as a scientific medical profession.

From the white mouse to *Homo sapiens*

How did the medical profession receive the introduction of female sex hormones as a new type of drug? The clinical reports published in the *Nederlands Tijdschrift voor Geneeskunde* gave Organon's female sex hormone therapy mixed reviews. The results of the clinical trials in the 1920s fell short of the high expectations that had accompanied the marketing of the new drug. At an international congress in 1927, clinicians reported poor results in clinical trials with female sex hormones. Most clinical trials undertaken in The Netherlands and abroad had given negative results. In 1929 the Dutch gynecologist Van Dongen judged the results of female sex hormone therapy as disappointing: "the route from the white mouse in the laboratory to *Homo sapiens* in the consulting-room is a long route that is not yet bridged" (Dongen 1929: 3,787). These poor results were blamed chiefly on the small amounts of active hormonal substance present in the commercial hormone preparations, and on underdosage in the prescription of female sex hormones.

The critical evaluation of clinical trials with female sex hormones indicated two strategies: to improve the quality of the products and to increase the dosage. Organon had anticipated this criticism and had already adopted both strategies. In advertising campaigns and clinical trials Organon suggested increased dosages,[11] and it introduced a new female sex hormone preparation under the trade name of *Ovariaalhormoon Folliculine Menformon*, advertised as "the first standardized female sex hormone" (usually referred to as *Menformon*).

In contrast to its earlier products, Organon had tested the activity of *Menformon* in animal experiments. With the use of standardized biological assays, the quantity of active substance in this female sex hormone preparation could be estimated (Organon Archive August 1926, undated letter). Organon evaluated the marketing of *Menformon* in a special issue of *Het Hormoon* published in 1956 to celebrate the thirtieth "anniversary" of this hormone preparation:

> thanks to Laqueur, among others, the first extensively purified and standardized – water-soluble – estrogenic hormone preparation was put on the market. This was a very significant occasion. Previously, ovarian preparations had been applied, but the unreliable activity of these preparations was a serious handicap. Clinical research and practice was henceforth provided with a preparation with which one could work more precisely, and from which more stable results could be expected, and it had also the major advantage that it could be injected.
>
> (HAWK 1956)[12]

At an international congress in September 1927, the quality of this product was judged much higher than the female hormone preparations from other countries, and the position of Organon was improved in the world market (Organon Archive 26 October 1927).

The close cooperation with Laqueur's laboratory once again proved its crucial importance for Organon.

Female sex hormones as universal drugs

The initial clinical trials in the early 1920s were mainly restricted to the treatment of menstrual disorders, in particular amenorrhea. By the late 1920s, female sex hormones were promoted for a substantially wider array of medical indications. This trend may have been facilitated by the marketing of Organon's new product *Menformon*, a less expensive drug available in larger quantities than the previous product.[13]

The first extension in medical indications consisted of the prescription of female sex hormones for menstrual disorders other than amenorrhea. In 1927, Laqueur advised the Dutch gynecologists involved in clinical trials to administer *Menformon* also to female patients with multiple menstrual bleedings (polymenorrhea) and in cases of very heavy menstruation (hypermenorrhea). Laqueur noted that if these trials succeeded, the indications for female hormone therapy could be increased substantially (Organon Archive 22 December 1927).

This extension to other medical indications is also reflected in Organon's publicity for female sex hormone preparations. In the first advertisement for *Ovarnon* in January 1925, medical indications were not described at all. The advertisement mentioned only that literature would be sent upon request. Evidently, knowledge of the therapeutic effects of female sex hormone therapy was too vague to formulate a well-defined description of medical indications.[14] But in a 1927 advertisement for *Menformon* (published in more than thirty countries), medical indications were described for the first time. Hormone therapy was now recommended for "all anomalies of ovarian function, causing disorders in menstruation and other sexual functions in women, in particular retardation in growth of the genital organs leading to sterility and in cases of menopausal complaints" (Organon Archive 28 September 1927).

In less than two years, the medical indications for female sex hormone therapy were thus extended from the treatment of menstrual disorders to the treatment of menopause, infertility, and problems of the genital organs. Although this extension of medical indications was quite substantial, female sex hormone therapy remained restricted to the gynecological clinic. This restriction disappeared after 1927, when Organon extended the clinical trials for female sex hormone therapy to the psychiatric clinic, thus creating an even broader market for female sex hormones. In December 1927 Organon initiated the first clinical trials in psychiatric clinics in Germany, in which female sex hormones were administered to female patients for treatment of schizophrenia and melancholia (Organon Archive 22 December 1927). The prescription of female sex hormones in cases of psychoses and depressions attributed to disorders in the menstrual cycle was also described (Beek 1933; Esch 1935; Organon Archive 19 August 1933).

In 1929, female sex hormone therapy was further extended to other medical indications. In the pamphlet advertising *Menformon* to Dutch and British general practitioners, Organon not only mentioned gynecological and psychological disorders, but also included dermatological diseases (such as eczema) and diseases of the joints; both disorders were presumably related to the dysfunction of the ovaries. Other medical indications mentioned in reports from Dutch and German gynecologists, general practitioners and psychiatrists on the results of female sex hormone therapy in female patients, suggested an even wider therapeutic use: for epilepsy, hair loss, eye disorders, diabetes, hemophilia and even chilblained feet (Organon Archive 19 August 1931, 7 October 1932, 28 January 1933, 30 April 1934, 20 May 1934 and 13 February 1935).

This wide range of therapeutic applications illustrates how, since the 1920s, female sex hormones developed from a treatment specifically indicated in cases of well-defined menstrual disorders to a more universal medicine applicable for a wide variety of conditions in female patients, all attributed to dysfunction of the ovaries. Medical practice in the United States shows a similar pattern in the application of female sex hormones. By 1933 the *American Council on Pharmacy and Chemistry* described this practice in female sex hormone therapy:

> Theelin [the name American scientists used for female sex hormones] and related preparations have been used in practically all the special ills the human female is heir to.
>
> (Anonymous 1933)

Female sex hormones as specific treatment for menopausal and menstrual disorders

Organon was, however, not satisfied with the broadened and unspecific applicability of female sex hormones. As late as 1932, Laqueur complained that a well-defined clinical picture for female sex hormone therapy was still lacking (Organon Archive 13 April 1932). Organon and Laqueur therefore initiated large scale clinical trials to investigate more thoroughly the therapeutic activity of female sex hormones. In the 1930s, the organization of (for the time) large-scale clinical trials was no longer curtailed by the high prices of hormone preparations during the 1920s.

In 1932, Laqueur approached the director of the women's clinic of an Amsterdam hospital in order to conduct a clinical trial in 100 female patients, according to the methodology of double-blind trials.[15] He hoped to investigate the effects of female sex hormones in female patients with a complex of symptoms attributed to the menopause, such as high blood pressure, increased heart rate, headaches and psychological depression. The idea that menopausal symptoms could be treated with female sex hormones was not new. At the turn of the century menopausal complaints had been the major indication for treatment with ovarian preparations. But such treatment had become discredited because gynecologists were not satisfied with its results (Dongen 1929: 3,781–3,782). Laqueur again suggested female sex hormone therapy for the treatment of menopausal women, expecting better results with the new preparations. To conduct these trials, Laqueur requested that Organon distribute female sex hormones free of charge. Gynecological clinics in Austria were also requested to conduct large-scale clinical trials on patients with menopausal symptoms (Organon Archive 14 September 1932).

In addition to large-scale clinical trials, Laqueur also enlisted the cooperation of a health centre in Amsterdam specializing in the treatment of rheumatism and other kinds of physical diseases, the Institute for Physical Therapy. The cooperation with this institute illustrates vividly the manner in which Organon tried to direct female sex hormone therapy as a specific treatment for women in the menopause. Specifically, in 1937, Laqueur approached the Institute for Physical Therapy to conduct clinical trials with female sex hormones in exchange for free hormone supplies from Organon. Laqueur convinced Organon to give hormone preparations free of charge by suggesting that this institute provided an excellent place for large-scale trials which would result in scientific publications from which Organon would benefit (Organon Archive 23 February 1937).

In organizing the trials, Laqueur's laboratory played an intermediate role between Organon and the institute. One of Laqueur's collaborators at the Pharmaco-Therapeutic Laboratory, the biologist John Freud, was also in charge of the organization of the trials. Freud visited the institute regularly and advised the medical staff about cases in which hormone therapy would be appropriate. Subsequently, Freud reported his advice to Organon and requested the free delivery of the required hormone preparations (Organon Archive 23 February 1937).

The institutional context of this cooperative venture directed female sex hormone therapy toward the treatment of middle-aged women. These patients had previously been treated with physical therapy. The introduction of female sex hormones thus offered a new therapeutic treatment. In 1937, Laqueur summarized the clinical trials in the Institute for Physical Therapy:

> If one evaluates the cases in which the health centre has asked for endocrinological advice, it is striking that until now exclusively female patients have been indicated, and that 50 per cent of these cases consisted of women in the menopause with illness of the joints and obesity.
>
> (E. Laqueur 1937)

The hormonal treatment of these patients gradually extended from a specific therapy for obesity and rheumatism to a therapy for other diseases in elderly women. Women visiting the health centre for treatment of specific complaints were also treated for other symptoms ascribed to menopause, thus providing a wider array of medical indications for female sex hormone therapy (Organon Archive 2 November 1937).

In the 1930s, many diseases of older women were increasingly attributed to low levels of sex hormones during the menopause. Because low levels of sex hormones were defined as a "deficiency" of sex hormones, symptoms previously not defined as illness became subject to medical intervention.[16] The cooperation of Organon and the Pharmaco-Therapeutic Laboratory with the Institute for Physical Therapy reflects on a small scale this broader construction of the menopause as a hormonal deficiency disease that can be treated with female sex hormones. In 1931 the German gynecologist, Bernhard Zondek, introduced a hormonal typology of menopause, suggesting a division into three periods, each characterized by a specific hormonal excretion, correlated with specific clinical symptoms: the polyhormonal phase (characterized by a large excretion of female sex hormones in the blood), the oligofolliculin phase (characterized by a decrease in female sex hormone production) and the polyprolase phase (characterized by a large quantity of gonadotropic hormone) (Hoeven 1931).

In the late 1930s, Organon promoted the treatment of menopause as one of the major indications for female sex hormone therapy. In 1938 the board of directors of Organon decided to choose menopause as the major medical indication in the yearly advertisement campaign for female sex hormone preparations. At this meeting, Organon emphasized that, in addition to these advertisements, it would be extremely important to achieve the acceptance of female sex hormone therapy as a specific treatment for menopausal symptoms by the Health Financing Institution (Organon Archive 8 December 1938). The board of directors decided to approach the management of the major Dutch industries with large numbers of female employees, for example Philips, Hero and Jamin, to inquire about the seriousness of the menopausal complaints of their female employees. In its strategy to convince the Health Financing Institution of the relevance of female sex hormone therapy for menopausal symptoms, Organon based its arguments on the economic relevance of treating the large number of women employees of menopausal age. In this manner Organon used the economic interests of others in promoting its own economic advancements. The construction of the menopause as a hormonal deficiency disease was thus also directed by economic motives (Organon Archive 19 October 1938).

In addition to the menopause, in the 1930s female sex hormone therapy also became more specifically focussed on menstrual disorders. In 1931, Marius Tausk proposed that Laqueur should initiate large-scale clinical trials to investigate the function of *Menformon* in menstrual disorders. Tausk suggested contacting the Dutch Council of Labor to initiate clinical trials in industrial companies with large numbers of female employees (Organon Archive 6 October 1931).[17] These clinical trials served a double purpose. In addition to obtaining more systematic results on the clinical relevance of female sex hormone therapy, these trials also functioned as a major vehicle in promoting female sex hormones as the specific medical treatment for menstrual disorders.

Moreover, in the early 1930s the hormonal definition of menstruation was extended to include psychological aspects attributed to hormonal changes during the menstrual cycle. In 1931, the American gynecologist Robert Frank introduced the diagnostic category of "premenstrual tension," a period preceding menstruation with symptoms including fatigue, a general feeling of tension, irritability and lack of ability to concentrate. Frank ascribed these symptoms to the increased activity of female sex hormones during this period of the menstrual cycle (Frank 1931: 1,053–1,057)

This reconstruction illustrates how, in the 1930s, female sex hormone therapy was promoted as a specific treatment for disorders in menstruation and menopause. The medicalization of menopause and menstruation opened up an enormous market: almost all women for many years of their lives.[18] The promotion of female sex hormone therapy as a specific treatment for menstruation and menopause, however, did not change its image as a much more widely applicable treatment. In the late 1930s, female sex hormones were still being prescribed for a wide range of indications. In the *Pocket Lexicon for Organ and Hormone Therapy* (published in 1937) Organon recommended female sex hormone therapy in as many as 34 out of 129 indications listed in this lexicon, a rather exceptional practice compared to the applicability of other organ and hormone preparations (Anonymous 1937).

Contraception and pregnancy

Reflecting on the wide range of medical indications for female sex hormone therapy, it is striking that hormonal control of reproduction did not develop into one of the therapeutic uses of female sex hormones until the 1950s. This is even more remarkable if one considers the fact that female sex hormones were applied as a medical treatment to regulate the menstrual cycle. The possible application of female sex hormones as contraceptives, however, did not go totally unnoticed. In 1933 Samuel de Jongh, one of Laqueur's collaborators, advised Organon to introduce *Menformon* as a contraceptive. The response of Organon to this proposal was rather apprehensive. Tausk suggested that contraception was a very difficult subject in The Netherlands, and advised de Jongh to approach the British birth control clinics. Tausk also considered approaching a Dutch gynecologist, but decided, after discussing the matter with Laqueur, not to promote the introduction of *Menformon* as a contraceptive. Although Organon did not adopt his suggestion, de Jongh continued to discuss the contraceptive possibilities of female sex hormones. In 1935, in the Dutch journal *Acta Breva Neerlandica*, de Jongh recommended the use of *Menformon* as what we now know as the "morning-after-pill."[19] He described the use of *Menformon* for this purpose during the period between coitus and the time of the next expected menstruation.[20]

Contraception as a medical indication for female sex hormone therapy was not further explored in clinical trials or research in The Netherlands. In other countries the subject of hormonal contraception seems to have been explored to a considerably greater extent than in The Netherlands. In Austria as early as 1920, the gynecologist Ludwig Haberlandt had emphasized the significance of "hormonal temporary sterilization of women for medical practice and social and sexual hygiene." In 1930 Haberlandt, in cooperation with an Austrian pharmaceutical firm, introduced the first hormonal contraceptive. Dutch gynecologists evaluated this means of contraception very critically, particularly because of the risk of complete infertility (Pinkhof 1931: 99). Although the possibility of birth control by means of the safe period method was discussed in Dutch medical journals, the idea of developing specific hormonal contraceptives was not mentioned (Organon Archive 12 December 1932).

In this case, the negative attitude of Dutch clinicians, general practitioners and the pharmaceutical industry with respect to birth control constrained the development of research on the use of female sex hormones as contraceptives. Dutch gynecologists generally opposed birth control, arguing that contraceptives – not only hormonal contraceptives but also contraception in general – were a threat to women's health and the cause of all kinds of gynecological complaints (Snoo 1940). Although after the First World War the issue of birth control had evolved into a major social topic, promoted in particular by a prominent middle-class movement in the United States, and Britain, as well as The Netherlands, the subject of birth control did not become integrated into the research agenda of reproductive scientists.[21] After the first World Population Conference held in 1927 in Geneva, "research in reproductive biology was intensified and additional funds became available for specific projects." These projects, however, did not include research on contraception. In spite of these efforts, American, British, and Dutch researchers "turned to the study of other aspects of reproductive physiology." Nor were American pharmaceutical companies engaged in contraceptive research. Although there existed a mass market, the moral and political attitude toward contraception constrained the introduction of hormonal contraceptives. Because of these constraints "the subject of birth control was not taken up again until after World War II" (Borell 1987: 51–87; Clarke 1987a: 130).[22]

In contrast to contraception, pregnancy did become one of the major issues in sex endocrinology. Sex endocrinologists provided the clinic with a specific test to detect pregnancy by means of analysis of the hormone content of the urine of (pregnant) women. In 1928, the gynecologist Bernhard Zondek and the chemist Selman Ascheim, both working at the Charité hospital in Berlin, introduced the first laboratory test for pregnancy, based on bio-assays in animals, a test that became known as the Ascheim-Zondek test.[23] This test had the major advantage of detecting pregnancy at a much earlier phase than the classical gynecological techniques (Tausk 1978: 42). Following the example of a German pharmaceutical industry advertising this pregnancy test, Organon decided to include this test in its research program. In 1936 Tausk reported to Laqueur that

> The pregnancy test is included in our routine research and on request we can include the analysis of urine samples without any effort. . . . It has always been our policy to perform these tests free of charge for patients who cannot afford them. In this way, we mean to use the pregnancy test as propaganda.
>
> (Organon Archive 26 September 1937)

Although Organon had excluded the prevention of pregnancy from its agenda, the prediction of pregnancy became one of its routine diagnostic assays in the late 1930s.

THE PROMOTION OF MALE SEX HORMONES

Early expectations and clinical trials

The first standardized preparation of male sex hormones was not put on the market by Organon until 1931, five years after the equivalent drug for women. Since 1924, Organon had been marketing an organ preparation made from testes (*Testanon*), but it was not standardized by biological tests. The relative delay in marketing a standardized preparation was caused mainly by technical problems in finding appropriate assay-methods for standardization and (as we have seen) in gaining access to the required amounts of raw materials.

Remarkably, the decision to develop standardized male sex hormones as an Organon product seems not to have been as self-evident as for female sex hormones. Before Organon decided to start production, Tausk had to be convinced by Laqueur of the commercial value of this product. Organon had serious doubts about the therapeutic activity of male sex hormone preparations and decided to market male sex hormone only under the condition that the clinical effects should be known in advance. Laqueur disagreed with Tausk on the necessity of clinical trials before marketing male sex hormones, and argued that "it is not the task of a pharmaceutical industry to retain the marketing of a much requested product" (Organon Archive 2 July 1930).

Technical problems further delayed the actual marketing of the first standardized male sex hormone preparation. The major problem was how to produce a highly purified hormone preparation free from other substances of similar solubility, and in particular free of female sex hormones. We saw before how, to the astonishment of many scientists, male urine and testes, applied as raw materials for the production of male sex hormones, contained not only male sex hormones but also substances defined as female sex hormones (Organon Archive 2 June 1930).

In the mean time, Laqueur initiated preliminary, small-scale clinical trials, delivering male sex hormone preparations to some of his clinician acquaintances in university clinics, both in Berlin and Amsterdam, with whom he had collaborated earlier. In January 1931, Organon started selling the first standardized male sex hormone preparation under the trade name of *Hombreol* (Organon Archive 3 December 1930).

What were the early expectations concerning the therapeutic value of male sex hormones? And to whom did Organon expect to sell its new product? In contrast to female sex hormones, the marketing of male sex hormones was not characterized by high expectations. On the contrary, both laboratory scientists and Organon were apprehensive. The modesty of these claims can be understood from what had happened earlier when a scientist had promoted therapy with testes preparations. Charles-Edouard Brown-Séquard had ruined his reputation by claiming rejuvenation and the revival of sexual activity in elderly male patients following the use of testes preparations (Corner 1965: iv). In the 1920s, Brown-Séquard's claims again revived. The controversial claims about testicular therapy were not confined to the last decade of the nineteenth century but continued into the early decades of the twentieth century. Practitioners in France and the United States began to transplant monkey (and other) testes into men and animals, a practice that came to be known as "the monkey gland affair." Similar to the early testes extracts therapy, this gland transplantation became a subject of public debate and controversy in the 1920s. This controversy was even greater and more lasting than that surrounding Brown-Séquard. The testicular transplantation practice lasted through 1930 when the surgery gradually began to lose credibility.[24]

To avoid a negative association of its products with these earlier speculations, Organon initially promoted male sex hormone therapy for a totally different and very specifically described indication: the treatment of hypertrophy of the prostate. Marius Tausk described this expectation in 1932 in *Het Hormoon*:

> A disease which, by its origin, makes one think of the causal role of an insufficient hormone production, is hypertrophy of the prostate. The fact that this disease always develops later in life legitimizes in every respect the presumption that a shortage of testis hormone plays a role in this. Whether this is correct, only the clinic can prove, by trying to affect this disease with standardized preparations. More than with any other hormone, in this case the necessity arises from a close cooperation between the clinician, the experimentor, and last but not least, the technician.
>
> (Tausk 1932a)

This restriction directed the promotion of male sex hormone therapy to urologists. The urologists were acquainted with the medical treatment of prostate hypertrophy. The major advantage of hormonal treatment of prostate hypertrophy was obvious. If male sex hormone therapy turned out to be successful, it could replace surgical intervention as the only possible treatment for this disease (Tausk 1933). This type of indication was in particular propagated by Laqueur. In 1934 Laqueur evaluated the clinical trials in cases of prostate hypertrophy in *Het Hormoon* as very promising, indicating that two-thirds of the cases had shown remarkable improvement (Organon Archive 27 October 1930; Tausk 1934a: 25–29).

The promotion of male sex hormones as specific drugs for the treatment of prostate hypertrophy was received rather favorably. In the late 1930s Dutch urologists published only positive reports, urging general practitioners to use male sex hormones:

> I would not fail to impress on you once again not to deny your prostate hypertrophy patients the chance to be relieved from their misery in a simple way.
>
> (Capellen 1936)

In 1937 Laqueur's colleague de Jongh concluded that the treatment of prostate hypertrophy, initiated in The Netherlands, had developed as one of the major indications for male sex hormone therapy in many other countries (Jongh 1937: 49).

Male menopause

Although much criticized, the early experiences with testes preparations also suggested another application of male sex hormones: the treatment of sexual disorders, like impotence and loss of libido, in particular in elderly men (Organon Archive 13 February 1931). This indication is also described as the *climacterium virile*, the male menopause.[25] Organon did not, however, put much effort into promoting hormonal treatment of these menopausal symptoms in men. They did not initiate clinical trials in order to test the therapeutic effect of male sex hormone therapy for the treatment of impotence and libido problems. This can partly be understood from the lack of an institutional context in which clinical trials could be organized. In the 1920s, the taboo on sexuality still constrained men with sexual problems from seeking medical care. Men with prostate hypertrophy would eventually ask for medical care; but older men with impotence seldom visited the general practitioner or the clinician. Moreover, sexological clinics did not yet exist in the 1930s. Organon's advertising policy reflects this apprehensive approach. Although by 1937, hormonal treatment of men with impotence and libido problems had developed into one of the major medical indications in Germany, Laqueur persuaded Organon to emphasize instead the treatment of prostate hypertrophy (Organon Archive 8 May 1937). Laqueur argued that emphasis on sexual impotence in advertising male sex hormones was far too risky because of the negative connotations with the claims of Brown-Séquard (Organon Archive 19 October 1938). The ghost of Brown-Séquard was apparently still very much alive in the late 1930s, and so were gland transplant surgeries. This restriction by Organon in advertising its male sex hormones seems to have been confined specifically to The Netherlands. In Britain, Organon advertised sexual impotence to the same extent as prostate hypertrophy (Figure 5.3).

Although heavily criticized by Laqueur, Organon decided that this type of advertising was quite appropriate for Britain, because of the different mentality of British general practitioners, who were not likely to object to such advertisements (Organon Archive 21 November 1939). In addition to these cultural constraints on the hormonal treatment of impotence, the therapeutic relevance of this treatment was also criticized (Organon Archive 13 May 1937). Many scientists as well as clinicians emphasized the psychological character of impotence and libido problems.

A third indication suggested for male sex hormone therapy were psychological disorders, such as depression, melancholy and schizophrenia (Organon Archive 17 November 1932; 11 October 1933). In 1931 Laqueur advised Organon to place *Hombreol* at the disposal of psychiatrists in order to implement clinical trials (Organon Archive 10 March 1931). These clinical trials seem to have taken place only on a small scale.[26] This indication, in particular schizophrenia, was also handled with the utmost

"A. man aged 60 complained of impotence

". . . He was a thoroughly healthy man with increased subcutaneous fat on his breasts, abdomen and buttocks . . . After a preliminary course of injections . . . potency was regained . . . and local inunction of an ointment was started.

"Apart from the maintenance of sexual function, the most obvious effects have been the new growth of hair and an increase in virility enabling this patient of 60 to play 36 holes of golf without undue fatigue."

See "Percutaneous Absorption of Male Hormone"
Lancet, 3rd December, 1938, p. 1284

NEO-HOMBREOL
Testosterone propionate
Ampoules and Ointment

Adequate supplies continue to be available

ORGANON LABORATORIES LTD.
77 NEWMAN STREET, LONDON, W.1

Temporary Address: 22 Parkwood Avenue, Esher. Telephone: Emberbrook 4058

Figure 5.3 Advertisement for Neo-Hombreol in *The Lancet* that was not used in the promotion campaign for male sex hormones in The Netherlands.

care. In discussing this hormone therapy for schizophrenia with Organon's pharmaceutical industrial partner in Britain, Laqueur was advised that pharmaceutical companies should not arrange clinical trials because psychiatrists were skeptical and could be won over to hormone therapy only if the pharmaceutical industries did not push too hard:

> There must be, of course, a number of psychiatrists intent on finding an organic basis for schizophrenic disorders, and it would be nice to have them buy their therapeutic material from us; but perhaps this is more likely to happen if we do not arrange a clear-cut experiment.
>
> (Organon Archive 30 November 1935)

In contrast to the female menopause, the medical attention given to the male menopause, which was characteristic of the last decade of the nineteenth century, gradually diminished during the early decades of the twentieth century. Here we see how the pre-idea that virility is controlled by the male gonads gradually disappears from the forefront in sex endocrinology. The scientific community distanced itself quite clearly from the earlier claims on male hormones, promoted by scientists like Brown-Séquard and Steinach. This does not mean that the idea that virility can be affected by male hormones totally disappeared. The idea is kept alive in more popular writings on sex hormones, exemplified in *The Male Hormone*, that strongly advocates the use of testosterone for evoking "eternal manhood" (Kruif undated). This shift in focus from male menopause to female menopause can be understood in the context of professionalization that took place in the medical sciences at the turn of the century. To demarcate the boundaries between the medical profession and the flourishing paramedical practice, clinicians increasingly opposed clinical quackery. The pharmaceutical company anticipated the reservations of the scientific community toward this use of male sex hormones in its endeavor to become accepted as a science-based industry. In this process, early claims in the treatment of aging men with testes preparations and glandular implants, gradually passed into the realm of quackery.

Male sex hormone therapy as a specific treatment for prostate hypertrophy

In contrast to female sex hormones, the marketing of male sex hormones was not immediately successful. In 1931 Laqueur complained that the selling of *Hombreol* did not show any progress and advised Organon to supply free preparations to leading Dutch general practitioners. The reason for the disappointing sales was sought in the poor quality of this product, which had led to negative results in clinical trials. To solve this problem, Laqueur's laboratory and Organon put more effort into improving the quality of male sex hormone preparations. Scientists found the answer ironically in making hormone preparations from a combination of both male and female sex hormones. In contrast with the earlier problems in producing male sex hormone preparations (in which scientists removed female sex hormones from the raw material to prepare purified male sex hormone preparations), scientists now added female sex hormones to male sex hormone preparations in order to improve their therapeutic activity. In 1931, Laqueur advised Organon to organize large-scale clinical trials with combined preparations of male and female sex hormones: *Hombreol Menformon*. The prescription of this new product was mainly indicated in cases of prostate hypertrophy and psychological disorders, such as depression and melancholy.[27] In 1937, Organon put a new hormone preparation on the market under the trade name of *Testosteron*. In contrast to the other male sex hormone preparations, this hormone was prepared from testes instead of urine. The successful isolation and chemical identification of testosterone in Laqueur's laboratory in 1935 faciliated the synthetic production of male sex hormone preparations, thus making available for therapeutic purposes much larger and less expensive quantities of male sex hormones. In 1936 Dutch urologists were approached by Laqueur to participate in the organization of clinical trials (Organon Archive 18 December 1936). A review of the medical literature in *Het Hormoon* in 1938 indicates that the synthetically manufactured testosterone esters (testosterone acetate and testosterone propionate) were used on a wide scale in the late 1930s (Tausk 1938b).

In sum, male sex hormone preparations were promoted mainly as a specific therapy for prostate hypertrophy and more tentatively for sexual and psychological disorders. Following the dualistic paradigm of sex endocrinology, the clinical use of male sex hormones was restricted to men. Emphasis on prostate hypertrophy as the major indication is evident in Laqueur's request in 1930 to the Ministry of Defence to obtain permission to collect male urine in military barracks. Laqueur explained the relevance of collecting male urine:

> It is rather likely that male sex hormone preparations affect a whole series of symptoms of old age in men, not only sexual functions, and also bring about favorable effects in a psychological sense. I envisage in particular the therapeutic treatment of prostate hypertrophy, one of the most serious geriatric complaints in men, which is possibly related to the absence of adequate male hormone.
>
> (Organon Archive 14 October 1930)

The indication of prostate hypertrophy was also emphasized in Organon's negotiations with the Health Financing Institutions to obtain funding for male sex hormone therapy (Organon Archive 19 October 1938).

The reception of male sex hormone therapy shows vast national differences. An inquiry among German urologists, surgeons, neurologists, dermatologists and general practitioners in 1937 illustrates that prostate hypertrophy and sexual and psychological disorders were indeed the three major indications for male sex hormone therapy. The same inquiry also indicates that the medical practice of male sex hormone therapy in Germany was much more varied than in The Netherlands, including dermatological disorders, anomalies in the development of genital organs and the stimulation of beard-growth (Organon Archive 20 April; 8 May 1937). In the United States the medical profession was rather critical of the promotion of male sex hormones. In 1939 the Council on Pharmacy and Chemistry published an evaluation of male sex hormone therapy in the *Journal of the American Medical Association*:

> Within the past few months extravagant claims for the action of the male sex hormone testosterone have appeared in professional and lay publications ... it is the Council's belief that many claims for it have been grossly exaggerated.

The council considered hormonal treatment as successful only in cases of absent or atrophic testes, or in cases of undescended testes:

> all other claims are either exaggerated or immature and should be disregarded until substantial evidence becomes available on which to evaluate them.

> (Council on Pharmacy and Chemistry 1939)

In The Netherlands, male sex hormones did not develop into a widely applicable treatment, as did female sex hormones. In the *Pocket Lexicon of Organ and Hormone Therapy*, Organon recommended male sex hormone therapy in only 3 of 129 indications in which treatment with hormone and organ preparations was advised (Anonymous 1937). Compared to female sex hormones, Organon's marketing strategy for male sex hormones was modest. Organon's propaganda was restricted to advertising campaigns and did not include asking industrial companies to test hormone therapy among their male employees, as had been done to promote female sex hormones.

CRACKS IN THE SCIENTIFIC AND THERAPEUTIC PROGRAM

In the original theory, sex hormones were conceptualized as chemical agents that were strictly sex specific in origin and function. Following this conceptualization laboratory scientists, pharmaceutical companies and gynecologists made two types of sex hormones: male and female. As we saw in Chapter 2, the sexual specificity of sex hormones became a topic of debate during the 1920s and was gradually abandoned. How did this crack in the scientific program affect sex hormone therapy?

From an evaluation of the therapeutic uses of sex hormones it is clear that the idea of a sex-specific function directed the therapeutic application of sex hormones, particularly throughout the 1920s and the early 1930s.

The clinical trials as well as the prescription of female sex hormones was restricted exclusively to women. Male sex hormones were prescribed only to men. Although this dualistic approach dominated the therapeutic use of sex hormones, the crack in the paradigm did not leave the clinic untouched. From the early 1930s, the first indications gradually emerged for "paradoxical" hormonal treatment, as the prescription of female sex hormones to males and vice versa was named. W. Petterson, a general practitioner in Berlin, evaluated this development in hormone therapy in 1933:

> The recognition of the fact that the living organism, male as well as female, is bisexual in disposition, gave rise to the introduction of paradoxical sex hormone therapy. Until recently, it was an established fact that in the man only testis hormone and in the woman only ovarian hormone was therapeutically effective. The application of het-erosexual sex hormones, whether or not in combination with homo-sexual sex hormones, has recently been shown in interesting cases, particularly with respect to chronic skin diseases. These reports led to critical discussions. Notwithstanding all this, scientists were not inclined to investigate experimentally this remarkable and obviously paradoxi-cal reaction.
>
> (Petterson 1933)

Such "paradoxical" hormone therapy came in particular to be applied in diseases ascribed to an "endocrine imbalance": a "deficiency" in male or female sex hormone (Petterson 1933: 716). In the 1930s, *Menformon* was prescribed to men in cases of specific eye diseases (retinitis pigmentosa), prostate cancer and disorders in the vascular system (Organon Archive 17 April 1937). Testosterone was prescribed to women for indications similar to those of female sex hormones, in particular menstrual disorders, psychological disorders and menopause (Tausk 1939a). "Paradoxical" hormone therapy seems to have been directed to women to a much greater extent than to men (Novak 1939). Although the use of sex hormones was no longer strictly sex specific, the model of sex specificity remained the dominant approach in the clinic. The crack in the scientific program led only to minor changes in the therapeutic program. In the *Pocket Lexicon of Organ and Hormone Therapy*, Organon mentioned "paradoxical" hormone therapy explicitly in just one out of thirty-seven indications in which the prescription of female or male sex hormones was advised. In 1938, Marius Tausk reviewed the practice of the prescription of male sex hormones to women as "very remarkable," but concluded that

> although treatment with testosterone resulted in a striking improve-ment, this treatment will certainly not replace the known hormonal therapy of menopause with ovarian hormone![28]

In this manner, clinicians and pharmaceutical companies further reinforced the concept of sex hormones as two separate entities: male sex hormones as new drugs particularly for men, female sex hormones as new therapy for women.

Another crack in the research and therapeutic program appeared when studies were published suggesting that the use of female sex hormones might lead to cancer. In 1932, Lacassagne, a zoologist at the Radium Institute in Paris, reported the induction of carcinoma in experiments with female sex hormone injections into male mice. Since the 1930s, an assumed relation between female sex hormone therapy and cancer had been debated intermittently (Tausk 1934b). The first reactions of Organon to these publications were rather moderate. In 1934, Tausk reviewed these reports in *Het Hormoon*, concluding that there was no risk involved in the therapeutic use of female sex hormones (Tausk 1934b). In 1936, Organon acknowledged, however, possible negative effects of these publications for the promotion of female sex hormone therapy. In discussing the publicity campaign for a new female sex hormone preparation (*Dimenformon*), Tausk and Laqueur emphasized that the introduction of a preparation that could be used in smaller dosages had a 'strong propagandistic effect with respect to the actuality of the carcinogenic question' (Organon Archive 7 December 1936). Following the publicity of the French pharmaceutical company Crinex, who had organized a wide-scale propaganda campaign against the use of concentrated female sex hormone preparations because of the risk of cancer, Organon decided in 1937 to circulate a special brochure on female sex hormones and cancer (Organon Archive 12 August 1937). In 1939, Organon reassured the medical profession that the risk of cancer was not very serious. Citing Laqueur's colleague John Freud, Tausk suggested in *Het Hormoon* that

> for fear of unpleasant consequences, one should not use anything for therapy or for food. One does not forbid kitchen salt just because one kilogram, taken at one time, may cause a deadly toxication.

Tausk concluded that the use of female sex hormones in therapeutic dosages would not cause cancer (Tausk 1939b: 127).

The introduction of the first synthetic female sex hormone, preparation DES (diethylstilbestrol), once again fueled the debate over the carcinogenic character of female sex hormones. In 1939, reports were published of breast cancer following injections with stilbestrol. The debate on the carcinogenicity of female sex hormones scarcely affected the promotion and reception of female sex hormones. The medical profession, as well as the pharmaceutical industry, emphasized their positive experiences with female sex hormone therapy.[29]

CONCLUSIONS

This story of hormonal drugs illustrates in a lively way that the development of a drug does not stop the moment it appears on the market – that is just the beginning. The marketing of sex hormones included the continuous testing of hormonal preparations in both the laboratory and the clinic. At the moment this story begins, sex hormones were merely chemical products with a largely unknown therapeutic value and an unexplored market. Sex hormones may best be portrayed as drugs looking for diseases.[30] Before the actual process of marketing could begin, the pharmaceutical company had first to create its audiences. It was clear that Organon could succeed in creating a market only if it linked up with the needs of the medical profession: the company had to create arrangements with the medical community in order to find diseases that could be treated with its new products. The only strategy to become informed about the therapeutic value of sex hormones was the organization of clinical trials.

These clinical trials played an important role in establishing the relationships between laboratory scientists, pharmaceutical entrepreneurs and clinicians, with laboratory scientists as intermediaries between the pharmaceutical company and the medical profession. We saw how Laqueur mediated all contacts between Organon and the medical community. Laqueur, as both a laboratory scientist and a trained physician, was the ideal actor to bridge these two worlds. Laqueur managed to convince his colleagues of the benefits of cooperating with Organon by promising the provision of high quality hormonal drugs in exchange for the delivery of raw materials and their cooperation in clinical trials. Laqueur thus enabled Organon to get access to the required raw materials and to a context in which the therapeutic value of its new products could be defined.

Most importantly, clinical trials also functioned as major devices in linking drugs to their audiences. The trials enabled Organon to cultivate a loyal clientele in the medical profession, and they assured Organon of close ties to its market. These alliances with the medical community contributed greatly to the success of Organon as a hormone manufacturer. The contacts Laqueur mediated between Organon and the medical profession were of vital importance for the hormonal enterprise. Without the cooperation of the medical profession the construction of hormonal drugs would have failed altogether.

The story of hormonal drugs also illustrates that drugs must be considered as the embodiment of interests that become mutually defined through social networks. The final drug profile is not shaped by the interests of one specific actor, for example laboratory scientists, but by the interests of different groups of actors, both in and outside the laboratory. The adoption of this view enabled us to understand how the development of hormonal drugs focussed particularly on female sex hormones and women. The production and marketing of female sex hormones as "scientific drugs" matched the needs of both gynecologists and pharmaceutical entrepreneurs to establish their scientific status, an endeavor in which they were mutually dependent. Cooperation with the clinic provided the industry with the institutional context for the organization of clinical trials to negotiate the final drug profile for female sex hormones as a new class of scientific drugs. Moreover, the gynecological clinic provided the industry with an available and established clientele, with diseases that could be subjected to hormonal treatment. The promotion of female sex hormones fitted seamlessly into already existing institutional structures formulated earlier in the century as part of the professionalization of medicine and the rationalized organization of service delivery. Prior to the introduction of sex hormones, clinics and hospitals focused already on reproductive phenomena, thus providing the required institutional structures in which female sex hormones could flourish.[31]

This cooperation with industry provided gynecologists in turn with a new class of drugs that served their struggle to attain the status of "scientific medicine." In establishing its status as a scientific profession, gynecologists – and the medical profession in general – claimed to improve medicine, moving away from the earlier medical practice of "folk drugs" and "quackery." Sex endocrinology provided the gynecologists with the tools to delineate the boundaries between "quackery" and "scientific medicine." Laboratory scientists provided standardized measurement of hormones and standardized hormonal preparations that could be used in gynecologists' clinical research and practice. Gynecologists incorporated sex endocrinology into their research and practice because they believed that the theories and tools provided by the laboratory could help to make gynecology more scientific. The use of standardized tests and drugs held the promise "to produce data seemingly independent of the gynaecologists as well as the patients' subjective judgement. These sorts of technologies strengthened gynaecologists' claim to objective judgement" (Bell 1987: 537). In their striving for a scientific image, the clinic and the pharmaceutical industry matched each others' needs, a process in which female sex hormones became of mutual interest and gradually developed into big science and big business.

The same success story cannot be told about the marketing of male sex hormones. Although there existed a potential audience for male sex hormones, it was not embedded in any organized market or resource network. The marketing of male sex hormones lacked institutional contexts for both the production and promotion of male sex hormones, as it was not connected to any medical profession comparable with gynecology. Organon and Laqueur promoted male sex hormones mainly to general practitioners and urologists. This network, however, did not provide the required conditions for any systematic clinical trials. The urological clinic provided only a small clientele with a relatively limited area of medical indications, again when compared to the gynecological clinic. Medical treatment in the urological clinic was restricted to urological diseases and did not focus on any other diseases of the male body. Like the manufacture of male sex hormones, the marketing lacked an appropriate institutional context for the promotion of male sex hormone therapy.

These differences in institutional contexts had far-reaching consequences for women. In the 1920s and 1930s, the female body became the major object for hormone therapy. Female sex hormones became applied as universal drugs for a wide array of diseases in women. In this manner, sex endocrinologists constructed the image of the hormonal woman: it was the female body that became increasingly subjected to hormonal treatment. Compared to women, the introduction of sex hormones had rather minor consequences for men. Although endocrinologists created a market for male sex hormones, male sex hormone therapy was introduced for only a relatively small number of medical indications.

The selection of drug profiles was profoundly shaped by cultural norms regarding masculinity and femininity. The pharmaceutical industry and the medical profession anticipated these norms, making the development of certain applications of hormones as drugs more likely than others. This is particularly clear in the promotion of hormones as drugs for male menopause and contraception for women. Laqueur deliberately dropped the hormonal treatment of the male menopause and the development of hormonal contraceptives from his agenda because he was afraid that the association of sex hormones with these types of medication might endanger Organon's scientific image. In this respect there are striking similarities between the issue of male menopause and female contraception. Involvement with these cultural, controversial issues did not enhance the legitimacy and professional authority of scientists. Scientists and clinicians who actually took part in studies of male menopause and contraception found themselves marginalized within the profession. These cultural constraints have molded reproductive sciences and technologies in Europe and the United States, although there seem to exist graded differences between the USA, Britain and mainland Europe. The cultural climate in Britain with respect to contraception and the male menopause seems to have affected scientific research in these issues to a lesser extent than elsewhere, a quite interesting observation that needs further analysis.

In summary, we can conclude that the marketing of sex hormones was profoundly shaped by cultural and institutional factors. In a context in which contraception and the male menopause were illegitimate subjects in medical science, and the physiology of the male reproductive system was not institutionalized as a medical specialty, sex hormones became marketed as specific drugs for menstruation and the female menopause, and not for contraception and the male menopause. These technological choices shaped the development of sex endocrinology in the following decades. The idea of hormonal regulation of the male menopause has not been taken up by the medical profession at all since the 1930s. The development of hormones into contraceptives was not taken up until the 1950s and 1960s. In the next chapter we follow the hormone researchers, the pharmaceutical companies and the medical profession in their final quest: the transformation of hormones into the contraceptive pill.

6 The transformation of sex hormones into the pill

Most people today will associate hormones with the pill. Hormonal contraceptives are indeed the most powerful outcome of the introduction of the concept of the hormonal body in the 1920s and 1930s. Although the possibility of using hormones as contraceptives was mentioned as early as 1921, it took three decades before scientists actually began to develop contraceptive hormones. When the pill eventually came into existence, it was greeted with enthusiasm. By the late 1950s and early 1960s, less than a decade after initial testing in animal studies, the pill was being consumed daily by millions of women all over the world. Never before in medical history had a medical technology witnessed such a rapid and broad diffusion (McLaughlin 1982: 38; Segal and Atkinson 1973: 350). "Probably the best indicator of its acceptance is the fact that we no longer use a capital *P* or inverted commas when writing about it, because everyone understands that the pill refers to only one kind of tablet," at least in the western industrialized world (Bromwich and Parsons 1990: 24)

The contraceptive pill was a novelty on the market for contraceptive methods at that time. It was the first physiological means of contraception. That is, it prevented pregnancies by intervening in the internal processes of the body, rather than by means of an extraneous device (Rock 1963: 168).[1] Contraception now might be achieved by taking an "aspirin-like pill that would be unrelated to sexual intercourse." Moreover, the pill was a novelty since it would be the first drug in the history of medicine given to healthy people for a social purpose (McLaughlin 1982: 120; Vaughan 1972: 51).

This chapter focusses on how hormones were made into contraceptives. How did scientists succeed in transforming hormones into completely new types of drugs? For, prior to the 1960s female sex hormones were mainly used as drugs for menstrual and menopausal dysfunctions. What kinds of actions were required to make hormones into the contraceptive pill? In order to understand the story of the pill we need to theorize about what actually happens to scientific artefacts when they not only get out of the laboratory but also get into a new generation. Constructivist approaches, again, may be helpful. Constructivists hold that scientists do not operate independently or outside a social or political context. They actively select and create the contexts in which their claims may be made relevant.[2]

This is exactly what happened in the case of the pill. In 1953, Gregory Pincus decided to develop a pharmaceutical product for one specific purpose: the control of fertility. Pincus thus chose to make knowledge claims about hormones relevant in a totally different context. This drastic change in the history of hormones may best be understood if we explore the activities that went into this recontextualization. I shall describe how the pill could be called into existence only if scientists redirected their work to other evidential contexts in which they could establish the required links between the technology-in-the-making and its new audiences and consumers. The successful transformation of hormones into contraceptives required a linkage to a world which was not yet inhabited by hormones: the world of birth control. By entering this domain, the story of hormones became entangled with big politics. The birth control arena was, and still is, a highly political world in which birth control ideologies mix with cultural imperialism. During the making of the pill, the story of hormones turned into a very dramatic one in which Caribbean women became the guinea-pigs of one of the most revolutionary drugs in the history of medicine.

I begin with a brief history of how the development of contraceptives became an issue on the research agenda of endocrinologists in the early 1950s. Next I analyze in detail the clinical trials and field trials in which hormones were made into contraceptives. In contrast with the previous chapters, this chapter deals particularly with research and development activities in the United States. The pill was developed in the United States, not in Europe. The dominant position of European scientists and pharmaceutical firms in the field of hormones, characteristic for the 1920s and 1930s, was broken in the mid-1940s by the newly established Syntex Corporation. This American firm introduced a much simpler and cheaper production process based on the use of plant raw material, thus replacing the more expensive and time-consuming practice of using human and animal materials (Gelijns 1991: 161; Maisel 1965: 43–58).

BIRTH CONTROL: FROM TABOO TO TECHNOLOGY

When scientists took up the testing of hormones as contraceptives in the early 1950s, it was not an entirely new topic on their research agenda. The possible use of hormones as agents to control fertility was mentioned as early as the 1920s. The first publication mentioning hormonal contraceptives can be traced back to Austria. In 1921, the gynecologist Haberlandt described the results of experiments in which he transplanted the ovaries of pregnant rabbits and guinea-pigs into animals which were not pregnant. The animals became temporarily sterile. The author added that this "sterilization method" could perhaps be applied to women by the administration of extracts from the ovaries of pregnant animals (Vaughan 1972: 9). The idea of hormonal contraceptives was first discussed in public at the Seventh International Birth Control Conference held in Zurich in 1930 (Borell 1987: 83). At this time, however, it was hardly more than a theoretical debate. The nature of the substances which had to be taken to achieve contraception in women became clearer only when the first sex hormones were isolated and synthesized. In 1937, Makepeace, Weinstein and Friedman, three scientists from the University of Pennsylvania, were the first to test a hormone, progesterone, for its contraceptive activity. They described the effects of giving progesterone to rabbits: the ovaries of these rabbits did not release any egg cells (Makepeace *et al.* 1937). The first synthetic progesterone was developed in 1939 as a reaction to the growing interest in this hormone as a drug for the treatment of several reproductive disorders in women, a development that I described in the previous chapter (Vaughan 1972: 7, 9).

Despite these developments, the paper on what came to be known as "the inhibiting effect" of progesterone on ovulation failed to trigger research by others. Research on hormonal contraceptives gradually waned in the late 1930s, due to a complex set of factors (Borell 1987). The Second World War partly accounts for the lapse in research activities. Pincus, the "father" of the pill, described in *The Control of Fertility* how the special demand of war research accounted for a shift in interest toward studies of adrenocortical function, particularly in relation to physical and mental stress (Pincus 1965: 5). Moreover, birth-control research was not very popular in the 1930s because there was a widespread prohibition against any applied research by university or research institute based scientists. In the United States as well as in Britain, scientists who opted for applied research were often pushed into less prestigious jobs (Clarke 1985). This situation continued even into the 1950s. In the United States "there were perhaps a half a dozen or maybe a dozen people working on clinical testing of any contraceptive methods in the mid 1950s. They were largely denigrated as being in the pay of pharmaceutical companies" (Jaffe in Anonymous 1978: 61–62). There were other constraints that also shaped the field of contraceptive research from its early years until the late 1960s, including the political and moral taboo on sexuality, and on birth control in particular. In the United States federal and state laws prohibited the dissemination of contraceptive information, including contraceptive devices until well into the 1960s.[3] The controversial status of any research that might be associated with contraception has had important consequences in terms of scientific recognition and access to research funding.[4]

Major American funding agencies such as the National Institute of Health and the National Science Foundation would not fund basic research in the reproductive sciences at a level equal to that for research on other major organ systems. The National Institute of Health was even forbidden from funding birth control research prior to 1959.

(Clarke 1990b: 20, 27)

The funding of reproductive research thus depended largely on private initiative (Ingle 1971: 236).

The few reproductive research projects that actually did take place in the 1930s focused on improving fertility rather than restricting fertility. In the words of one of the American endocrinologists of that period:

We have not been trying to develop fertility control. We have been trying to improve fertility primarily, up until very recently at any rate. All through the thirties the object was to improve fertility. . . . It has not been, I'm sorry to say, a real objective of the biological sciences, endocrinology, to develop birth control hardware.

(Greep in Anonymous 1978: 10)

The impetus for change of this restrictive political and scientific climate came from three social movements: the birth control movement, the population control movement and the eugenic movement.[5] All three aimed to limit human reproduction by separating sexuality from reproduction. The birth control movement emerged as a feminist-inspired movement "to enhance women's control over their reproductive capacities" shortly after the turn of the century in the United States as well as in Europe. The eugenics movement, aimed at "improving" humankind by "applying agricultural breeding principles to humans," emerged in the 1880s. The population control movement, inspired by the Neo-Malthusian ideology, focused on control over the "numbers of people and their distribution in relation to the distribution of resources" (Clarke 1990b: 24).

After the Second World War these movements more or less "merged and consolidated under the banner of family planning and population studies" (Clarke 1985; Gordon 1976).[6] By the 1960s the fear of a "population bomb" threatening the social order became the dominant ideology of governments in the United States and Europe, drawing leading reproductive scientists gradually into solving "population problems" (Clarke 1990b: 21). In the USA the National Academy of Sciences and Public Policy "selected population problems as its focus in 1961" (Clarke 1990c: 13). The relationship between reproductive scientists and these social movements may best be portrayed as a love–hate affair. On the one hand, reproductive scientists attempted to distinguish their work from these rather controversial movements. On the other hand, they depended on them since these movements provided increasing support and legitimacy for reproductive research (Borell 1985).

The direct impetus to change the status quo in research on hormonal contraceptives came from two women: Margaret Sanger and Katherine Dexter McCormick. In 1951, Margaret Sanger, a women's rights activist and pioneer for birth control in the USA, accomplished her goal of getting scientists to work on the development of "a simple, cheap contraceptive."[7] She had lobbied extensively for years for "the creation of a laboratory program of contraceptive research" (Borell 1987: 53). Since the 1920s, Sanger had founded two journals to provide forums in which scientists could present their research findings about contraception (Christian Johnson 1977: 66). Her strategy to cooperate with scientists was intended to lend more prestige and legitimacy to birth control and to develop means of birth control better than the existing methods (Christian Johnson 1977: 65, 66). She faced major problems in mobilizing scientists for her project. Most scientists chose to work on theoretical rather than applied problems, and were reluctant to move into this type of research, afraid of becoming the subject of controversy (Christian Johnson 1977: 66).

In 1951, at the age of 68, Margaret Sanger finally succeeded in finding her scientist: Gregory Pincus (Pincus 1965: 67; Vaughan 1972: 24). Pincus, a biologist interested in endocrinology and reproductive functions, started his career at Harvard and had won worldwide recognition as a prominent researcher in the study of hormones.[8] Following a controversial publication on parthenogenesis in 1937 he was denied tenure at Harvard and continued his career outside the university, and not without success. In the 1940s, with Hudson Hoagland, another Harvard reject, Pincus built a major research organization: the Worcester Foundation for Experimental Biology, a private, independent, non-profit research institution located within 40 miles of Boston with social and professional ties to Harvard and Boston Universities and the State Hospital of Worcester (Christian Johnson 1977: 70).

The major constraint on the Worcester Institute and Pincus in the early years was the continuous need for grants. Funds for research were not abundant in the 1940s unless one held a position at a well-supported university or research institute (Werthessen and Johnson 1974). Pincus, described by his colleagues as "a scientific entrepreneur in the best sense," "a scientist-statesman with great organizational abilities," succeeded in organizing the funds needed to finance the research institute (Vaughan 1972: 43–44) In the late 1940s, he contacted G.D. Searle and Company, a pharmaceutical firm that had already sponsored several other projects carried out by the Worcester Foundation, among others the development of anti-epileptic drugs. At that time Searle was reorienting its interests (Anonymous 1978: 31). Pincus persuaded the company to go into the hormone business. (McLaughlin 1982: 135–136; Ramirez de Arellano and Seipp 1983: 106).[9] He convinced them "that it is to their advantage to have basic research done at the Foundation, the cost of it, they could write it off and that in every case the projects engaged in might have practical significance."[10] Searle, increasingly interested in the potential of hormones for a variety of drug applications, supported Pincus's research with enough money to finance a staff of a dozen researchers at the Worcester Foundation. In the 1940s, the foundation's research agenda consisted of "the testing and screening of hormone compounds submitted by Searle for evaluation of properties relevant to eventual use as drugs for the treament of arthritis and other diseases" (Christian Johnson 1977: 70). Pincus functioned for many years as Searle's consultant for the development of hormonal drugs. Pincus's relationship with Searle thus shows remarkable similarities with the cooperation between Ernst Laqueur and Organon that has been described in previous chapters.

Before Margaret Sanger contacted him, Pincus had no particular interest in contraception (McLaughlin 1982: 97). In his own account of what made him decide to begin contraceptive research, Pincus refers to "two overtly ascertainable factors: a visit from Mrs. Margaret Sanger in 1951, and the emergence of the appreciation of the importance of the 'population explosion' " (Pincus 1965: 5). Sanger obviously convinced him of the necessity to develop hormonal contraceptives and, of equal importance, she provided him with the required funds.[11] She raised $150,000 mainly from her friend Katherine Dexter McCormick, to get Pincus started on research towards what she called a "universal contraceptive" (Seaman and Seaman 1977: 63). Thereafter McCormick, one of the first women graduates of the Massachusetts Institute of Technology, contributed a sizeable annual budget to support Pincus's work. Actually, she financed the entire research effort that brought the pill into being. Not a single penny of government money was invested in it (McLaughlin 1982: 93) nor was there money from Searle or other pharmaceutical companies. Searle was skeptical of the proposed project of testing hormones for contraceptive activity (Ramirez de Arellano and Seipp 1983: 106). They provided the hormonal compounds (described later), but not the money. The pill was thus born in the margins of the established medical academic institutions. Or as McCormick described it: "Personally I doubt if they, at Harvard, would ever have found an oral contraceptive!"[12]

This short history shows how hormone research was gradually reoriented toward contraception. Most importantly, it illustrates how the first step in this recontextualization of hormone research was initiated by feminist birth control activists, rather than by scientists themselves. Pincus decided to focus his research on the contraceptive potential of hormones only after he had met Margaret Sanger. Sanger and the birth control movement were crucial in making contraceptive research an issue on the research agenda and in creating the financial conditions for this research project. In the next section we follow Pincus to see how he tried to create the relevant contexts for the clinical testing of hormones as contraceptives.

TESTING IN DISGUISE

After Margaret Sanger's visit, Pincus began the search for the "universal contraceptive." In 1951, he took up the line of research that Makepeace and his colleagues had initiated in 1937: the effects of progesterone on ovulation. As a first step, Pincus had two of his staff members, the chemist Min-Chueh Chang and the biologist Anne Merrill, administer various amounts of synthetic progesterone to female rabbits to investigate the dosage and timing required to inhibit ovulation. They succeeded in duplicating the long-ignored Pennsylvania experiment and reconfirmed that progesterone could work as a contraceptive, at least in animals (McLaughlin 1982: 108).

The next step, testing the compounds' ovulation inhibiting potential in humans, could not be taken in the laboratory. For this Pincus needed a clinic. At a scientific conference in 1952, he happened to meet John Rock, a professor of gynecology at Harvard, with whom Pincus had collaborated on an earlier research project.[13] Rock, the director of the Free Hospital for Women, one of the busiest infertility clinics in the United States, was a major advocate of the application of hormone research to clinical gynecology (Reed 1984: 354). At this conference Pincus learned about Rock's clinical studies, in which he tested progesterone among his women patients for a purpose totally opposite from that of Pincus: the treatment of infertility.[14] The Free Hospital promised to be an ideal test site for Pincus's purposes. The hospital attracted many leading gynecologists and functioned as a private research clinic (McLaughlin 1982: 41). Despite their different missions, Rock and Pincus seemed to follow similar approaches. Actually, they were working on different aspects of the same problem – the manipulation of the process of conception – and they shared an interest in the same hormones (Rock 1963: 163). Cooperation between the laboratory and the clinic could be of mutual interest: it would provide Pincus with the required conditions for testing progesterone as a contraceptive in women, while Rock might profit from the cooperation since it promised a much broader investigation into the development of infertility drugs. Rock, who well knew the contraceptive effect of the treatment with progesterone (McLaughlin 1982: 110), accepted Pincus's request to extend his research on progesterone to the compound's potential use as a contraceptive.[15]

Pincus's animal experiments and Rock's clinical studies were a step forward in the search for hormonal contraceptives but nevertheless confronted them with a serious problem. Progesterone seemed to be more active if it was injected than if it was given by mouth. Pincus anticipated that injections were not suitable for a "universal contraceptive": women would not be in favor of repeated injections. Oral administration seemed a much more promising alternative (Christian Johnson 1977: 71; Vaughan 1972: 30–31). Pincus's animal experiments indicated that progesterone could be used as an oral contraceptive only in large doses, making it rather expensive. The making of an "aspirin-like" contraceptive required a synthetic progesterone that would be effective at a lower dosage, and thus cheaper to produce (Reed 1984: 355).

At this moment, a third actor appeared on the stage: the pharmaceutical industry. Pincus approached the major hormone-producing companies and asked them to send him samples of all the synthetic progesterones that they had manufactured (Maisel 1965: 12). Following this request, Pincus received nearly two hundred compounds, which were subsequently tested in his laboratory for their oral activity on "a small army of rabbits and rats" (Maisel 1965: 122; Ramirez de Arellano and Seipp 1983: 107) Initially, Pincus chose the products of two companies, Searle and Syntex, as the most promising oral progestins: compounds known as 19 nor-steroids.[16] Later he switched exclusively to Searle's product. As noted, Pincus already had strong alliances with the Searle Company in his role as scientific advisor and as screener of the firm's hormonal compounds. Rock was also acquainted with the firm, which had provided the required progestins for his infertility studies (McLaughlin 1982: 135–136). The delivery of progestins for the contraceptive research project further cemented the relationships between Pincus, Rock and Searle into a strong network of mutual dependencies. Both Pincus and Rock depended on the pharmaceutical company for the delivery of oral progestins. Searle, in its turn, required Pincus's laboratory and Rock's clinic for the organization of tests to decide whether 19 nor-steroids could be made into contraceptives. In this emerging network, Pincus was the pivot on which the other actors hinged. He mediated the contacts between Searle and Rock, transmitting Rock's findings to the company (Christian Johnson 1977: 75). Chang, who performed almost all the experimental work on oral progestins in Pincus's laboratory, characterized Pincus's role as follows:

> Without his wide knowledge of endocrinology, his organizational ability, and his good relations with the pharmaceutical industry as well as the medical profession, and above all, without his daring enterprise, all this work would be on the library shelves.
>
> (Vaughan 1972: 43–44)

The irony of this history is that these developments, which would eventually lead to the manufacturing and marketing of the first oral contraceptive, took place in Massachusetts, a state where rigid laws against birth control still functioned. As Rock put it:

> Life has a way now and then of mocking man's more questionable designs. It must have amused some citizens of the Commonwealth of Massachusetts, with its rigid law against birth control, to discover that the first breakthrough in contraceptive technology in 75 years suffered and survived its labor pains in the environs of Worcester and Boston.
>
> (Rock 1963: 159)

This restrictive climate, however, had an enormous impact on Pincus's and Rock's work: the testing of progestins as contraceptives can best be described as a testing in disguise. Rock's infertility studies turned out to be the ideal "undercover" strategy for the organization of clinical trials for the testing of the oral progestins that Pincus had selected in his animal studies. The contraceptive potential of their compounds could be tested in a research project designed for a totally opposite purpose: the stimulation of conception! Both Sanger and McCormick were enthusiastic about this location for the organization of the first trials on humans, very much aware of the fact that Rock's clinic provided a perfect "alibi" for research that clearly violated the law (McLaughlin 1982: 123).

The first testing of oral contraceptives thus took place as a parallel study in Rock's infertility studies. In 1953, Rock started a second series of clinical trials in which twenty-seven women were enlisted, all patients with infertility complaints drawn from the Free Hospital clinic, this time with the explicit aim of testing the trial compounds on ovulation (McLaughlin 1982: 115). The trials consisted of a rather extensive and complicated set of tests, all with the purpose of determining whether the trial compounds stopped ovulation. Rock's staff at the Free Hospital charted the length of the menstrual cycle and daily basal body temperatures, and also took daily smears of the vagina, a 48-hour hormone assay of the urine, and a monthly biopsy of the endometrium of the uterus (Rock and Pincus 1956: 892). In the clinic these trials were nicknamed the 'PPP,' the Pincus Progesterone Project, also known as the "pee, pee, pee project" because of the regular urine specimens that had to be checked (McLaughlin 1982: 117).

At Pincus's suggestion, the design of the trial was modified to adjust to the changed research goal. To quote Rock: "As a result of our discussions I instituted certain changes in our second series of 27 women" (Rock 1963: 163). One of these changes consisted of an adjustment in the regimen of taking the pills. Rock's infertility patients were quite distressed when they noticed that their menstruation ceased during the treatment with oral progestins (Maisel 1965: 119). If these women were distressed, Pincus and Rock reflected, it would be very likely that women taking progestins for contraceptive purposes would experience similar reactions. A contraceptive that suppresses menstruation did not meet the requirements of a "universal" contraceptive. Pincus therefore changed the medication. The pills should be taken for twenty days, starting on the fifth day after menstruation, as was the practice in the hormonal treatment of menstrual irregularities in the 1940s (McLaughlin 1982: 110).[17] This suggestion set the standard for the administration of progestins in all later trials and eventually for the use of the contraceptive pill in the 1960s.

The choice of this regime of medication was also shaped by moral objections to any drugs that would interfere with menstruation. Pincus was directly confronted with this norm by Searle's director of biological research, who let Pincus know that he did not want to take part in the development of any compound that might interfere with the menstrual cycle (McLauglin 1982: 111). In later publications both Pincus and Rock presented the effect of progestin on menstruation as a way of mimicking nature: women would still have their menstrual periods. In 1958, Pincus legitimized the regime of medication as follows:

> Actually, in view of the ability of this compound to prevent menstrual bleeding as long as it is taken, a cycle of any desired length could presumably be produced. We had chosen our standard day 5 through day 24 regime in the expectation that "normal" cycle length would occur.
>
> (Pincus 1958: 1,338)

Pincus and Rock emphasized that the pill was not "going against nature."[18] Or to quote Rock in recapitulating the development of the pill in 1963:

> Today, more than one million women of many countries are taking the pills, not simply because of their great effectiveness but also because they provide a natural means of fertility control such as nature uses after ovulation and during pregnancy.
>
> (Rock 1963: 167)[19]

This choice of the regime of administration exemplifies how medical technologies are modified to meet the needs of their users as well as moral attitudes toward intervening into nature.

The results of this first trial did not yet answer the question of whether the oral progestins could be made into the "cheap and safe" contraceptives that Sanger had envisioned. The women participating in this trial were after all suffering from infertility problems, and were not exactly the ideal subjects to test contraceptives. Rock and Pincus thought this test nevertheless informative. In their report in *Science* in 1956 they concluded:

> Despite adequate coitus, none of the 50 women became pregnant during the months of medication. Their long-standing infertility may make this zero figure of no import. Nevertheless, it seems of at least passing interest that within only 5 months of the last treated cycle, seven patients conceived.
>
> (Rock and Pincus 1956: 892)

Both Rock and Pincus felt that more clinical trials were needed. A single study of fifty and then of twenty-seven infertile women did not suffice to convince their colleagues. Actually, Pincus met severe criticism when he first presented their findings in public. At the fifth meeting of the International Planned Parenthood Federation (Margaret Sanger's brainchild) held in Tokyo in 1955, Pincus's presentation was received with yawns and skepticism. The tests used by Rock to check whether women had ovulated were criticized by other scientists as rather inconclusive (McLaughlin 1982: 121; Vaughan 1972: 36). With Rock's methods, the diagnosis of the incidence of ovulation could be assessed only by indirect testing. Clinical tests for a direct diagnosis of the suppression of ovulation, as against a diagnosable pregnancy, were not available (Clarke 1985; Rock *et al.* 1957: 326–327). The chairman of Pincus's session, Solly Zuckerman, professor of anatomy at Birmingham University, concluded at the end of the session:

> Promising though they may appear at first sight, I think it is fair to conclude that the observations reported by Dr. Pincus do not bring us as close as we should like to the goals of our researches.
>
> (Zuckerman as cited in Vaughan 1972: 36)

Reservations concerning possible side-effects of daily ingestion of the pill were uttered as well.[20] To quote Zuckerman again: "We need better evidence about the occurrence of side-effects in human beings. . . . There is an urgent need for prolonged observation before we draw any firm conclusions" (Vaughan 1972: 37). Rock, who had not accompanied Pincus to the Tokyo meeting, shared this opinion. Women participating in his trials had indeed complained of unpleasant side-effects.[21] To quote Rock:

> The none too positive assurance of the slightly uneasy experimenter was not entirely conducive to sublime confidence that all would be well. . . . In view of these results, it seemed advisable after 18 months to declare a short recess for renewed contemplation and appraisal.
>
> (Rock *et al.* 1957: 324)

This cautious attitude concerning possible risks for the subjects was not the only constraint delaying an extension of the trials to fertile women. Large-scale clinical trials for the explicit purpose of developing contraceptives were practically impossible to carry out since they would have violated the law. Rock and Pincus knew that legally they could not organize these trials at the Free Hospital without risking criminal prosecution in Massachusetts (McLaughlin 1982: 118).

Pincus considered an escape route: Puerto Rico, a location outside the continental USA. In Puerto Rico, laws prohibiting contraception did not exist at that time.[22] Pincus approached the dean of the University of Puerto Rico Medical School, who agreed to undertake the clinical trials. Neither Pincus nor Rock participated directly in the trial. The progestin study was carried out by one of Pincus's collaborators: Celso-Ramon Garcia, a Manhattan-born Spanish-American gynecologist. Rock functioned merely as medical advisor, personally examining the women's tissue samples, which were sent to him at his clinic in Brookline, Massachusetts (McLaughlin 1982: 118).

In Puerto Rico, Pincus kept on his guard as well. The trial was labeled a study of the effect of progestins on the menstrual cycle rather than a study of contraception (McLaughlin 1982: 118). Pincus did not under-estimate the political risks of his work. His colleague, Hudson Hoagland from the Worcester Foundation, has revealed how he and Pincus "used to get threats that we'd be killed" (Hoagland in Anonymous 1978: 49). Garcia described the political climate at that time as "so hostile that you couldn't get a physician in Puerto Rico to carry out any work." During the later field trials Garcia and his staff also received threats, particularly from the medical profession, including that "they would be barred from the hospital privileges, that they would be barred from taking board examinations, that they would be given every possible impediment if they collaborated any further with the programs in Puerto Rico" (Garcia in Anonymous 1978: 49).

This experiment in the clinic in Puerto Rico did not last long. The recruitment of volunteers was quite problematic. Most of the medical students dropped out, due to graduation and a reluctance to adhere to the troublesome requirements of the test: taking daily temperature and vaginal smears, collecting urine samples and submission to an endometrial biopsy. The trial included twenty-three women medical students, of whom only thirteen remained in the project for three months. Disciplining women to the rigorous conditions of the trials was obviously not an easy task. Pincus's correspondence shows that even the students who com-pleted the pilot-study "did not comply strictly with the demands of the experimental procedures." The student was held accountable for "irres-ponsible behavior" during the experiment, which would be held "against her when considering grades."[23] Garcia, after a vain attempt to recruit new students, then turned to female prisoners as potential subjects. These women, however, expressed objections to participation in the trial. The final setback for this Puerto Rican trial came when university officials learned about the contraceptive implications of the study and withdrew their support for the research project (McLaughlin 1982: 119; Ramirez de Arellano and Seipp 1983: 110).

After this débâcle in Puerto Rico, Pincus tried another escape route: a mental hospital. He approached the Worcester State Hospital, a mental institution located near his laboratory, with which he had cooperated in earlier experiments.[24] The hospital's director agreed to the organization of a clinical trial with fifteen patients, all classified as psychotics. The group consisted of seven women and eight men, the first (and last) male test subjects in the research project.[25] Despite the fact that the hormone preparations had a definite contraceptive effect in the male patients, men were not included in later trials due to the occurrence of side-effects. In this trial one subject was found to have smaller testicles after five months of taking progestin tablets.[26] Pincus met other constraints as well. The psychotic men did not exactly make easy subjects. The men's mental disturbances made it rather difficult to collect semen samples, one of the requirements for investigating the effects of progestin (McLaughlin 1982: 120; Vaughan 1972: 39, 40). The results of this trial, to put it mildly, did not give the decisive answer to Pincus's quest for the "universal contraceptive."

The restrictive political climate not only directed the choice of clinical testing locations, but also shaped the publication behavior of the scientists and clinicians involved in the project. The titles of the early publications do not inform the reader at all about the topic they are actually dealing with. All the papers published in this period bear rather misty titles, with neutral terms such as "progestins" and "menstrual cycle" as keywords. The first report that Pincus and Rock published in *Science*, for instance, is entitled "Effects of Certain 19-Nor Steroids on the Normal Human Menstrual Cycle". (Rock and Pincus 1956). In these early publications the authors only casually mention the inhibiting effect of progestins on ovulation, but make no claims about the possible use of progestins as contraceptives.

In this respect Rock, given his Catholic background and his reluctance to make any premature claims, seems to have acted more cautiously than Pincus. This was clearly the case at the conferences where they first presented their research. While Pincus had openly discussed the possible use of progestins as contraceptives at the conference in Tokyo in 1955, Rock avoided mention of it when he presented their research findings at the Thirteenth Laurentian Conference in 1956. He concluded only that: "We are led to suspect that ovulation has been inhibited in at least a very high proportion of the cases" (Rock *et al.* 1957).

This was a rather non-committal claim that had been made earlier by other scientists as well. Rock made no statement about the contraceptive potential of progestin. His audience, including representatives of the major hormone-producing pharmaceutical companies from all over the world, was clever enough to read between the lines. (McLaughlin 1982: 122; Tausk 1978: 387). In the concluding session, one of the conference participants remarked: "One fact which stood out in this study is that Dr. Rock has unwittingly given us an excellent oral contraceptive which may be employed with little untoward effect" (Rock *et al.* 1957).[27] The word was out that the Boston scientists and clinicians were on the track of a new contraceptive. It was clear as well that Pincus and Rock needed more substantial data to convince the scientific community of the success of their endeavor.

This episode of the making of the pill illustrates in a very lively way that Pincus's quest to find relevant contexts in which his claims about the contraceptive activity of hormones could be established was not an easy one. Initially, the selection of Rock's clinic seemed to be a perfect solution. The clinic provided Pincus with access to women who could be made into the first test subjects for the contraceptive-in-the-making. Pincus quite successfully reoriented Rock's research from conception to contraception. Nevertheless, Rock's clinic, and the other settings which Pincus selected, failed to provide the conditions for the testing of the contraceptive activity of hormones. The development of progestins into contraceptives required access to large groups of healthy, fertile women. Large-scale trials, however, could not be organized in the gynecological clinics of medical schools, since these trials were even harder to conceal than small-scale trials. Pincus and Rock had to create a testing location outside the domain of the established medical institutions. They needed a politically feasible location where the development of progestins into contraceptives could be put to the final test.

At this point, Pincus explicitly linked his research to the domain of birth control. He shifted his research activities from the gynecological clinic to the family planning movement. Pincus took refuge, again, in Puerto Rico, where the family planning movement had a widespread institutional base in the form of birth control programs and clinics. Or to summarize the situation in Garcia's words:

> The attempt was at first to go to the University of Puerto Rico and that's how I got involved in it. The attempt was to stay within a group of academic scientists. When that failed, then they went to seek out patients and the most logical place to find them was in the Planned Parenthood clinic.
>
> (Garcia in Anonymous 1978: 55)

AN ISLAND LABORATORY

The ultimate choice of Puerto Rico as the testing ground was shaped by a complex set of factors which illustrates the ways in which the development of new medical technologies takes place. Medical innovation requires the creation of contexts to establish the required links between the technology-in-the-making and its new audiences and consumers. If such a context does not exist, scientists have to create it. The making of the pill required the creation of what might best be described as "a laboratory in the field." The test location had to provide the same controlled conditions that were present in the clinical setting. It was quite clear that the field location had to meet specific requirements so that these trials would not fail altogether.

The prerequisite was that the location had to guarantee that women would not easily drop out of the project. But where could one find such a "cage of ovulating females," as McCormick bluntly put it (Ramirez de Arellano and Seipp 1983: 107)? In this respect an island seemed a perfect solution since its population tends to be rather stable. Pincus again opted for Puerto Rico, a "miniature world" which seemed to be an ideal location for the testing of progestins (McLaughlin 1982: 28).[28] The island's people were stationary, with hardly any opportunity to move elsewhere. Pincus's colleague Garcia explained the choice of Puerto Rico:

The basic aspect was trying to find an area where there were large numbers of fertile women that were in need of contraception; look, it was a question of the law of supply and demand and where you could carry out these studies under a close supervision of the individuals concerned. . . . The object was to set up a program in an area where you would have better control over the particular population that you are dealing with.

(Garcia in Anonymous 1978)

Pincus selected a location in one of the suburbs of the capital, San Juan, where large slum-clearance operations were being carried out, involving a new housing project. Many of the families who had just moved into these new houses had previously lived in hovels. This situation promised to minimize the risk that women would become lost to the continuous checks and examinations of the trials. Or, as Garcia put it:

The particular sites that were selected were the so-called Parcellas, the housing projects that were considered the elite amongst the indigent. They considered it a prize to have been selected to be living in those homes, in those apartments and therefore once they got into them, they never left. Their kids did but they didn't. And therefore we had the equivalent of a captive population which in the United States you would never have had.

(Garcia in Anonymous 1978: 66)

Puerto Rico thus promised to meet one major requirement of the laboratory. But an island in itself is, of course, not enough to make a "laboratory in the field." The development and introduction of new technologies requires an organizational infrastructure within which this testing can take place. Puerto Rico also met this requirement in the form of its Family Planning Association. In the early 1950s the family planning movement had a well-established base in Puerto Rico. The Family Planning Association, as the direct successor to the Population Association and other previous birth control organizations in Puerto Rico, was founded in 1953 and had inherited a widespread network of family planning workers and clinics. The aim of the association, continuing the work of previous organizations, was "to provide contraceptive services, stimulate interest in family planning, and carry out research concerning the efficacy and acceptibility of different birth control methods" (Ramirez de Arellano and Seipp 1983: 102, 128).[29] The association could rely on a well-trained and medically sophisticated staff. Because of its previous status as a US colony,[30] Puerto Rico had a well-developed university at its disposal, including a Medical School. The University of Puerto Rico, situated in San Juan, maintained frequent exchanges with the continental

American universities, facilitated by a direct air service between New York and San Juan (Ramirez de Arellano and Seipp 1983: 74). Celsio-Ramon Garcia, for example, who cooperated with Pincus and Rock in the progestin trials and founded the Department of Gynecology and Obstetrics at the Medical School of the University of Puerto Rico, received his training as a gynecologist at the State University of New York. (McLaughlin 1982: 118; Ramirez deArellano and Seipp 1983: 74). Consequently, the medical staff of the Family Planning Association was familiar with the "American approach," to use Pincus's words. The Puerto Rican Family Planning Association thus provided the local organizational infrastructure required for the testing of the progestins.[31] The medical profession did not show any interest in the trials of the new contraceptive. According to Garcia "the medical profession, the whole health care field in Puerto Rico, while it accepted and tolerated sterilization, just paid minor attention initially to the field trials that we set up in the Planned Parenthood organization" (Garcia in Anonymous 1978: 49).

A third requirement for creating "a laboratory in the field" was a population willingly available for examinations and interviews with the field trial staff. Where could women be found who would be motivated to participate in the trials? Again, Puerto Rico seemed very promising. Its colonial history had resulted in a well-established public health system. Puerto Ricans were thus accustomed to a reliance upon public health workers rather than family doctors (Maisel 1965: 128–129), a situation which might facilitate their participation in the progestin trials.

By choosing Puerto Rico as the test location, hormone research became inextricably intertwined with birth control politics. This choice clearly illustrates how scientists do not operate outside political contexts, but actively select these contexts. The making of the pill was an overtly politically inflected endeavor based on a very specific ideology concerning its potential users. In 1950, Sanger described this underlying ideology: "the world and almost our civilization for the next 25 years is going to depend upon a simple, cheap, safe contraceptive to be used in poverty stricken slums, jungles, and among the most ignorant people."[32] Sanger's expression reflects the then dominant ideology with respect to population control and economic development. After the Second World War, the problems of assisting what were then first identified as "underdeveloped countries" became of increasing international concern (Ramirez de Arellano and Seipp 1983: 88). In this period birth control was perceived as a prerequisite of development. Puerto Rico, given its status as one of the most densely populated and impoverished regions of the world, was considered a prototype underdeveloped country, right at the USA's doorstep (Maisel 1965: 129; Ramirez de Arellano and Seipp 1983: 88).[33] In the late 1940s overpopulation came to be considered as the basic cause of what was called the "Puerto Rican problem," with birth control as its major cure (Gordon 1976: 336).[34]

This population control ideology was shared by Pincus and Rock. In this respect the previous tests were not sufficient. Thus far the oral progestins had been tested only among a selected group of well-educated white women. These tests did not yet answer the question of how well educationally limited populations in Third World countries could be disciplined to take the pills regularly (Maisel 1965: 127). Consequently, Pincus and Rock sought a test location with a less-educated population than in the previous trials. Puerto Rico, whose population included a high proportion of semi-literate and illiterate women, met this need as well as the other requirements. Puerto Rico thus became the stage for testing the progestins.[35] It was on this island that Pincus and Rock began their final quest: the organization of field trials.

REPRESENTING WOMEN AS MENSTRUAL CYCLES

In February 1956, Pincus approached Edris Rice-Wray, medical doctor of the Associacion pro Bienestar de los Familias in San Juan (the Puerto Rican Family Planning Association) about the possibility of undertaking progestin trials in their birth control clinics. Rice-Wray, who held an appointment at the University of Puerto Rico and was medical director of the associacion as well as director of the US Public Health Field Training Center in Rio Piedras, seemed the ideal person to assist Pincus. She was experienced in the organization of family planning programs and had all the contacts necessary to gain access to possible test locations. Rice-Wray was willing to cooperate and agreed to supervise a series of prolonged field trials with Pincus's compounds that would be carried out under the aegis of the Family Planning Association. Rice-Wray was to be in charge of the fieldwork which included

> recruiting cases, distributing the contraceptive, monitoring the subject's reaction, and collecting the required data. Pincus and Rock retained control over the research design and provided facilities for laboratory and other analyses that could not be done in Puerto Rico.
>
> (Ramirez de Arellano and Seipp 1983: 113)

Pincus thus found everything he needed at the Family Planning Association.

The first field trial was organized in the new public housing development project in Rio Piedras. The superintendent of this housing project, who was sympathetic to birth control and a person familiar to the tenants, agreed to cooperate in the organization of the trial and provided Rice-Wray and her team with records of the families. She subsequently selected the first set of 130 subjects, all women who had previously been given conventional barrier contraceptives at the clinic of the associacion (McLaughlin 1982: 129; Maisel 1965: 130–131). The screening of women for the trial consisted of a complete physical examination, carried out by

Garcia, to ensure that the women were in good health (Maisel 1965: 131). Garcia also set up the meticulous data-keeping system (Garcia in Anonymous 1978: 47).

This test location seemed to be the right one. The women at Rio Piedras were eager to participate in the project, even to such an extent that Rice-Wray had to create a waiting list (McLaughlin 1982: 129). Many of these women had many children despite some use of other available contraceptives (Vaughan 1972: 49). The crucial question now was how these women could be motivated to participate in the trial for a longer period. All previous tests had been of short duration: no woman had taken the progestins for longer than a few months. The field trials had to answer questions about the effects of long-term use of the new contraceptive (Vaughan 1972: 41). The project would be successful only if women would not drop out too early. How could these women be turned into reliable producers of data?

The way in which the Rio Piedras trial was organized shows the strategies that Pincus and Rock used to discipline women to meet the requirements of their tests. The first requirement was that the women had to learn to follow the relatively complicated instructions of "one tablet a day, beginning on day 5 of the menstrual cycle until one vial of 20 tablets was consumed, i.e., through day 24 of the cycle" (Pincus 1958: 1, 335). Rice-Wray, in consultation with Pincus and Rock, assigned the responsibility to ensure a strict adherence to this regime of medication to a team of trained social workers. In the report of this trial, published in the *American Journal of Obstetrics and Gynecology* in 1958, Pincus described this regime:

> A schedule of visits by a trained social worker was arranged so that in every medication cycle each subject was seen shortly after she should have taken the last tablet. Initially only one vial was distributed to each woman. This was replaced on the social worker's visit. Since, in a number of instances, the housewives were not at home when she called, it was decided, after a few months, to leave two vials with each subject so that the continuity of the regime of medication (day 5 through day 24) might not be broken.
>
> (Pincus 1958: 1,335)

During the visits of the social worker, the women were asked to cooperate in interviews as well.

> At each consultation, information was elicited concerning the length of the menstrual cycle, the occurrence of side effects, the frequency of coitus, and the number of missed tablets. A rough check, in some instances, on the number of tablets omitted was made by counting those remaining in the vial.
>
> (Pincus 1958: 1,335)

This strategy to ensure that women would adhere to the required test protocols did not work in all cases. In the publications of this trial Pincus reported seventeen pregnancies due to what he described as "patient failure": these women had missed some days of tablet-taking (Pincus 1958: 1,335; 1959: 81).

Another, rather demanding requirement was that women had to submit themselves to regular physical examinations. Participants in the trial were expected to visit the Family Planning Association's clinic, or an affiliated physician, for a pelvic examination including a biopsy of the endometrium of the uterus, a vaginal smear, and a series of blood samples. At home they were expected to collect 48-hour urine samples. These examinations and tests were aimed at monitoring any harmful effects of the progestins on important organ systems (Pincus 1958: 1,335).

Disciplining women to submit themselves regularly to these examinations was not an easy task. For almost all the women the gynecological examinations were totally new. They were accustomed to seeing a doctor only when they gave birth (McLaughlin 1982: 131). In the 1958 publication of the Rio Piedras trial, Pincus was able to report only on a relatively small number of women actually participating in the physical examinations: the blood samples were carried out in thirty-nine women, the urine tests in forty-two women, and the endometrial biopsies, obviously even harder to acquire, were obtained only from "some of these subjects" (Pincus 1958: 1,338–1,341).

The hardest quest was, however, to ensure that the women would continue to participate in the trial. At this point the field trial in Puerto Rico turned out to be rather problematic. The original object was to enroll 130 women, but for various reasons participants kept dropping out (Pincus 1958: 1,335). In the Rio Piedras trial more than half of the women who started had withdrawn by the end of the year. Consequently, the trial did not meet Pincus and Rock's expectations. It was quite clear that more data were needed, not only to convince their colleagues but, even more importantly, to serve as evidence toward approval of the new drug by the Food and Drug Association (FDA) (McLaughlin 1982: 133).

Second and third trials were therefore quickly organized in Humucao, Puerto Rico, and a fourth one on another Caribbean island: Haiti (McLaughlin 1982: 133).[36] These trials suffered from the same handicaps as the first trial, although they showed a less dramatic drop-out rate of approximately 10 to 30 per cent (Pincus 1959: 8). Most women stopped the medication because of troublesome side effects they experienced during the pill-taking. Women participating in the trials had experienced unpleasant side-effects including dizziness, nausea and headaches, the most frequently mentioned complaints (Ramirez de Arellano and Seipp 1983: 116). In the first reports of the trials Rice-Wray therefore concluded that the pill "caused too many side-reactions to be acceptable generally" (McLaughlin 1982: 134). Pincus and Rock were also aware of possible adverse health effects of the hormones, particularly the growth of cervical, uterine or breast cancer. The participants of the trials therefore received regular physical examinations, including the vaginal smear test to screen for cervical cancer.

> These tests revealed no risk in the incidence of uterine cancer. . . . On the basis of these early studies the American Cancer Society and the Andre and Bella Meyer Foundation made substantial grants to finance even more extensive examinations among women participating in the Puerto Rican and Haitian field trials, studies which have continued over a period of more than eight years.
>
> (Maisel 1965: 139)

In order to check for the complaints of nausea and headaches, Pincus designed a test in which a group of women were given placebos. From this trial Pincus concluded that such complaints had a psychosomatic origin (McLaughlin 1982: 132). Other people involved in the trials attributed these reactions to the "emotional super-activity of Puerto Rican women" (Ramirez de Arellano and Seipp 1983: 116). Pincus ascribed the side-effects "to the small amount of estrogen that occurred in progestin as a contaminant" and requested the Searle Company to synthesize a compound that would be free of estrogen. Subsequent trials with the pure compound, however, showed an increase in the incidence of break-through bleeding. Pincus and Rock ascribed this to the missing estrogen and therefore decided to include this hormone again in the contraceptive compound. This combined estrogen-progesterone preparation was given the trade name *Enovid* (Ramirez de Arellano and Seipp 1983: 115).[37] Other reasons for dropping out were "moved or too distant, sterilized, separated from husband, disapproval of the husband, objections by the woman's own doctor, protests of the woman's priest" (Pincus 1958: 1,344). The contraceptive pill had to compete with other contraceptive methods, in Puerto Rico particularly sterilization. Many women who dropped out of the clinical trials chose sterilization as "a more desirable solution to the problem of fertility control" (Ramirez de Arellano and Seipp 1983: 134). Keeping women in the trial turned out to be a hopeless task. In sum, after three years of trials all the original subjects had been replaced by other participants. Or, to quote Pincus: "We try to watch them as best as we can and we attempt to regain the withdrawals for our research. Actually, we reach approximately 20%".[38]

Pincus and Rock addressed the problem of drop-outs that could not be solved in the field in their reports. Here we see how scientific reports are not simply a reflection of the proceedings of research, but are a far stronger tool than that: they are a representation that creates a new reality. Let us take a closer look at what happened in Pincus and Rock's reports. In most of their publications the women participating in the trials have disappeared completely from the stage. They were replaced, quite simply, by the number of treated menstrual cycles. In the 1958 publication of the Rio Piedras trial, Pincus concluded: "In the 1279 cycles during which the regime of treatment was meticulously followed, there was not a single pregnancy" (Pincus 1958: 133). And the 1959 publication in *Science*, describing all four Caribbean field trials, reported:

> We have recently collected and analyzed the data (to November 1958) from these four projects and present here the outstanding findings derived from these data; 830 subjects took the medication for a total of 8133 menstrual cycles, or 635 woman years.
>
> (Pincus 1959: 81)

A popular writer adopted this representation strategy as well. In *The Hormone Quest* the author concludes:

> By 1960 1600 women at the Caribbean Field Trial Centers had used *Enovid* as a contraceptive for from a few months to nearly four years. Their experience, as a group, with the new steroid covered nearly 40,000 menstrual cycles or – as medical statisticians prefer to put it – about 3000 woman-years of exposure to the possibility of pregnancy.
>
> (Maisel 1965: 134)

This representation strategy had important consequences. The very act of representing women as menstrual cycles resulted in a major increase of scale: the grand totals of the trials now included much more impressive numbers than a focus on the individual subject might have achieved. The trials were thus presented as having met their purpose: the testing of the progestins on large numbers of women over longer periods, as a prerequisite for its approval as a safe and reliable contraceptive.

THE CONTINUOUS TESTING OF THE PILL

The way in which the oral progestins were finally approved as contraceptives is a rather intriguing story. Based on the Rio Piedras trial and a handful of small-scale clinical trials in the continental USA, the FDA approved *Enovid* in 1957, not as a birth control pill but only as a treatment for menstrual disorders. According to Garcia this was a political choice:

> The first application was not as an oral contraceptive but as a gynecological agent to treat menstrual aberrations, and that was done with political calculation and it wasn't done with any other thing in mind because the contraceptive properties of it were well-known at that point.
>
> (Garcia in Anonymous 1978: 60)

Many actors understood very well what the FDA approval actually meant. In McCormick's words:

Of course this use of the oral contraceptive for menstrual disorders is leading inevitably to its use against pregnancy – and to me – this stepping stone of gradual approach to the pregnancy problem via the menstrual one is a very happy and fortunate course of procedure.[39]

In May 1960, the FDA eventually granted its approval for the marketing of *Enovid* explicitly for contraceptive purposes (Maisel 1965: 142). Pincus and Rock's representation strategy turned out to be successful. The FDA executives used both the results of the clinical trials and all the studies, "every page of them," from the Puerto Rican and Haitian field trials.[40] The Caribbean trials functioned as an important ingredient in convincing the FDA, the medical profession and health officials of the "universal" character of the new contraceptive: it was proven that it could be used by women of any color, class and educational background.

Following FDA approval, the new contraceptive could be put on the market. G. D. Searle and Company, very much aware of the novelty of the product and its potential to damage the company's reputation, did not take any risks. Its executives developed a careful marketing and public relations campaign. Ahead of the launching date for the product, they approached the editors of the *Saturday Evening Post* and *Reader's Digest* and negotiated three major articles, telling the story of "the new contraceptive that was being tested in Puerto Rico." This strategy was chosen to test whether their new product might generate any protest. The expected angry letters to the editors, however, did not appear. Searle had obviously misjudged the situation. Times were changing during the years that the pill was being developed. Despite the fact that contraception was technically a forbidden subject in Massachusetts, the moral attitudes to contraception and sexuality in general were relaxing in the 1960s (McLaughlin 1982: 137–138; Vaughan 1972: 52–53). Actually, by late 1959, half a million American women were already taking *Enovid*, originally prescribed to them as a drug for menstrual disorders, as contraceptives. Both doctors and patients knew the pill's contraceptive power well before it was marketed as such. The FDA, in its first approval of *Enovid*, had "mandated Searle that the drug would carry a warning to the doctors that women would not ovulate while taking the pills," a mandate which worked like a "free ad."[41] A similar practice existed in European countries. In The Netherlands a combined estrogen–progesterone preparation was first marketed in 1962 for the treatment of menstrual irregularities, carrying a warning that women would not become pregnant while taking this medication. This strategy was chosen to anticipate possible protests from physicians, the media, the lay public, as well as the mainly Catholic production personnel of Organon, the firm that introduced the pill to the Dutch market (Haspels 1985: 20). In Spain, this cautious attitude was even found up until the 1980s. "The Spanish Pharmacopoeia described estrogen–progesterone combinations as effective in regulating menstrual cycles, but as having the serious side effects of preventing pregnancy" (Veatch 1981). This practice exemplifies how the activity of a drug is not dictated by nature, but is the result of a socially conditioned selection process, in this case religious and moral attitudes toward birth control (Bodewitz *et al.* 1987).

Searle soon witnessed the profits from its "daring decision" to market *Enovid* as a contraceptive: the company's shares doubled in value in the years following FDA approval (Seaman 1969: 179). Other American drug companies, such as Syntex and Parke-Davis, did not take this risk. They felt that contraceptives were not a suitable business for an ethical firm (McLaughlin 1982: 137). Parke-Davis in particular was afraid that the marketing of a contraceptive would ruin their market in the Roman Catholic areas (Anonymous 1978: 36–37) The market, however, was more than ready to accept the new contraceptive.

The FDA's approval of the first oral contraceptive had an immediate impact on the health care system in the US. In the spring of 1960, many health department directors and welfare officials began to plan the opening of new contraceptive clinics (Maisel 1965: 216). The acceptance of *Enovid* as an officially approved drug did not mean, however, that testing had come to an end. Research and development of the new contraceptive remained a major issue on the research agendas of Pincus and Searle, and those of the many other scientists and companies that now joined the bandwagon.

Since the 1960s, field trials of *Enovid* and other related compounds have been continued and expanded. One of the problems to be solved, which would remain a major issue for further testing until well into the 1980s, was the proper dosage of the drug. The dosage used in the early clinical and field trials was merely guesswork, "a shot in the dark," as one of Pincus's colleagues described it (Vaughan 1972: 48). Systematic studies of reductions of the dose, needed to make the contraceptive "physiologically safer, but also more economic" (Pincus *et al.* 1962: 440) were not included in the early trials. This might have increased the risk of pregnancies, thus lowering the "success" rate of the medication, which was measured only in terms of non-pregnant cycles. After FDA approval was obtained, new trials were organized to give more serious consideration to the side-effects that continued to be reported by women and physicians, the most important of which was the risk of cancer (Ramirez de Arellanoa and Seipp 1983: 123).

The development of a pill with reduced dosage levels was taken up when the new contraceptive came to be used regularly by a great many women, underlying the necessity of producing a pill that required less raw material and that would cause fewer side-effects. A second generation of oral contraceptives under the brand name of *Ovulen*, with one half and later one-quarter of the dose of *Enovid*, was tested and put on the market in 1963. This first made the pill available outside the USA: in

Britain, Austria and South Africa. The third generation of the pill, available in the 1990s, contains a dosage that is only one-tenth of the progesterone and one-third of the estrogen levels of the first generation of oral contraceptives (Maisel 1965: 195, 201; Vaughan 1972: 49). The use of hormones as contraceptives since the early 1960s can therefore be described as an "infinitely large unofficial field trial" including women all over the world (Maisel 1965: 146).

CONCLUSIONS

This episode in the story of hormones illustrates how scientists reoriented the hormonal enterprise to a totally new purpose: the control of fertility. As I indicated, medical innovation can only be successful only if scientists succeed in selecting and creating the required contexts in which knowledge claims can be established. In this respect, the development of hormones into contraceptives faced serious constraints, which shaped the entire development trajectory, from the search for the required test locations to the enrollment of women in the trials, and from the approval of the FDA to the eventual marketing of the contraceptive pill. The pill was a novelty since it was a compound to be prescribed for healthy women. This meant that the organization of clinical trials could not easily follow the routines of other clinical testing. Trials for the testing of drugs to cure a specific disease could rely on patients who could be assessed in clinical settings. For the pill, such patients did not exist. The testing of the pill required "healthy patients" who did not suffer from any particular disease and consequently did not belong to the clientele of a specific clinic.

The search for the required test locations was highly constrained by the political and moral taboos on birth control. The major quest was therefore: where to find test subjects and a politically feasible test location. Due to these constraints, the history of testing the pill reads as a detective story in which the participants try to conceal their real intentions from anyone who might hinder their endeavor. In this respect, the first trial in which hormones were tested in humans speaks volumes: the contraceptive potential of the hormones was tested first among women who were being treated for infertility problems! Subsequent trials were organized in settings where only very specific groups of subjects could be assessed: a mental hospital, a medical school and a women's prison. These trials were not very successful in enrolling women. Established medical institutions could obviously not provide the required infrastructure for the development of the contraceptive pill.

What all this implied was that pill researchers had to create the required contexts themselves. The quest for "healthy patients" could be solved only by removing the tests to a completely different location: the infrastructure of the family planning organizations, particularly the Family

Planning Association in Puerto Rico. This displacement did not necessarily imply a preference for Puerto Rico. It is very likely that the required test location might as well have been found among family planning clinics in those states of the US continent that had no laws prohibiting birth control activities. Actually, one such trial was organized, in Los Angeles, at about the same time that the third trial in Puerto Rico took place.[42] The choice of Puerto Rico must therefore be understood as a mixture of cultural imperialism and practical testing considerations. Since the contraceptive pill was called into existence mainly because it was considered a technological fix for the population problem in "underdeveloped countries," its testing required a population that reflected this ideology: poor, illiterate women. Puerto Rico, with its poorly educated and impoverished population, provided such a testing ground.[43]

The hormone story thus evolved into a highly political story which clearly shows the crass manipulatory strategies of big politics which can ignore other communities. This is very different from the intimate involvement of the communities I described in the previous chapters, where there was a kind of see-saw of dominance that kept everyone very aware of whom they were dealing with.[44]

The displacement of the clinical tests from the medical institutions to the clinics of the family planning organizations had enormous consequences in terms of the women who eventually became the major test subjects for the contraceptive pill. The first large-scale trials, with all the risks involved, did not take place among the white majority of Americans or Europeans. It was Caribbean women who entered this history as the guinea-pigs of one of the most revolutionary drugs in the history of medicine. Obviously, women do not have the same position as "objects of scientific inquiry." This means that we cannot continue to address women as a group if we focus on knowledge production about the body. This conclusion is in line with the postmodernist approach in women's studies, which suggests that the feminist preoccupation with the category of woman tends to obscure and mystify the vast differences among women's experiences and characteristics in different cultural settings. Black feminists specified this claim by suggesting that feminist studies should take into account the differences between women that are created by the social contexts of being black or white.[45]

Applying this theoretical notion of the construction of differences to the story of the pill shows a rather peculiar pattern. The choice to test progestins in Caribbean women could be made only because scientists did not assume a priori fundamental bodily differences between women. All women are equal in scientists' theories on the role of progestins in reproductive functions, even to such an extent that scientists make women disappear from their reports altogether. We saw how, in publications about the pill, women who participated in the trials are replaced by menstrual cycles: woman is represented as "cycle." This representation strategy enabled scientists not only to make the most of their results, but also emphasized the similarities between women. The use of such categories as "cycle" replaces the individual subject by the group, suggesting a continuity that did not exist in the trials. That suggestion simultaneously affirms continuity while obscuring discontinuity by framing new scientific categories for data measurement. A representation in terms of cycles implies an abstraction from the bodies of individual women to the universal category of a physical process.

The history of the pill thus reads as the intriguing story of how scientists tried to construct similarities between women. This construction of similarities was not just a matter of discourse. During the testing of hormones, similarities were literally created by the introduction of a specific regimen of medication. As I indicated, Pincus could have made a menstrual cycle of any desired length by changing the prescription of how to use the tablets. He chose to make a "normal" menstrual cycle that subsequently became materialized in the pill. This diminished the variety in menstrual patterns among women: all pill-users have a regular four-week cycle. The pill thus literally created similarities in women's reproductive functions.

This emphasis on similarities was a prerequisite for the quest to develop a universal technology: a contraceptive that was meant to be used by women of any color, class or educational background. This dream of making the ideal contraceptive for any woman, regardless of her specific background, was not fulfilled. The main acceptance of the pill has been among middle- and upper-class women in the western industrialized world, with one major exception: China. Most women in Third World countries have adopted sterilization and intra-uterine devices as means of contraception (Seaman and Seaman 1977: 76). Despite the development of the pill, the problem of fertility control is not yet solved. Even in the 1990s, there still exists a large and unmet need for fertility control among women worldwide (Hardon and Claudio-Estrada 1991).

7 The power of structures that already exist

Science, more than any other investigative and descriptive activity, creates and conceals the contexts from which it arises.

(Duden 1991c: 20)

We need the power of modern critical theories of how meanings and bodies get made, not in order to deny meanings and bodies, but in order to build meanings and bodies that have a chance for life.

(Haraway 1989a: 580)

My argument throughout this book has been to show that sex hormones are not just found in nature. My concern was with finding an alternative explanation for the idea that the emphasis on the female body in hormone research simply reflects a natural order of things. *Beyond the Natural Body* illustrates how scientific body concepts such as the hormonal body assume the appearance of natural phenomena by virtue of the activities of scientists. In this archeology of the hormonal body I tried to unravel both the construction and the impact of this new understanding of the body. It is time to summarize and evaluate the major conclusions that can be drawn from my examination of the history of sex hormones.

MAKING THE BODY NATURAL

Since its introduction in the early decades of the twentieth century, the hormonally constructed body concept has gradually developed into a dominant mode of conceptualizing the body, even to such an extent that we are encouraged to assume that the hormonal body is a natural phenomenon. But what exactly is required to transform a scientific concept into a natural phenomenon? I suggest that an answer to this question can be found in one of the distinctive features of science and technology: its striving for universal, decontextualized knowledge. Scientific concepts attain the status of natural facts in a twofold process. First, scientists create the contexts in which their knowledge claims are accepted as scientific facts and in which their technologies can work. Scientists adopt what I would call a "(re)contextualization strategy" in which their knowledge claims can gain momentum. Second, scientists then conceal the contexts from which scientific facts and artefacts arise, in a process which I will refer to as a "decontextualization strategy."[1] One of the reasons why science succeeds in convincing us that it reveals the truth about nature is that the social contexts in which knowledge claims are transformed into scientific facts and artefacts are made invisible. Science makes us believe that its knowledge claims are not dependent on any social context. During the development of science and technology the established links with the worlds outside the laboratory are naturalized. "There was, or so it seems, never any possibility that it could have been otherwise" (Akrich 1992: 222).

The quest for universal knowledge

Let us first look more closely at how scientists have tried to create contexts in which their knowledge claims about sex hormones could be transformed into natural facts. The history of sex endocrinology shows both successes and failures, which can best be understood in terms of the notion of networks of knowledge. In this perspective, knowledge "never extends beyond and outside practices. It is always precisely as local or universal as the network in which it exists. The boundaries of the network of practices define, so to say, the boundaries of the universality of medical knowledge" (Pasveer 1992: 174). The successes and failures in scientists' striving for universal knowledge are thus related to the extent to which they are successful in creating networks. Bruno Latour's metaphor of the railroads exemplifies this point:

> When people say that knowledge is "universally true," we must understand that it is like railroads, which are found everywhere in the world but only to a limited extent. To shift to claiming that locomotives can move beyond their narrow, and expensive rails is another matter. Yet magicians try to dazzle us with "universal laws" which they claim to be valid even in the gaps between the networks.
>
> (Latour 1988: 226)

In terms of this network perspective, the concept of sex hormones was a strong concept because of its pronounced connotations for sex and the body. Female sex hormones could be linked with "female diseases" and related medical institutions, and male sex hormones to "male diseases" and related medical professions. The concept of sex hormones simultaneously summarized and simplified the interests of specific groups. At this point, however, there existed vast differences between knowledge claims about female sex hormones and male sex hormones. The previous chapters have shown how the networks that evolved around statements about female sex hormones were much more extensive and substantial than the networks around male sex hormones.

First, there were major differences in the number of researchers who became involved in both types of research. Because methods as well as research materials for female sex hormones were well developed and easily available, more and more researchers became involved in research on female sex hormones. We saw how the number of publications on female sex hormones increased steadily in the 1920s and 1930s and soon outnumbered those on male sex hormones.

Second, there were striking differences in the number and variety of the groups outside the laboratory that became involved in research on female and male sex hormones. Knowledge claims about female sex hormones could be linked rather easily to relevant groups outside the laboratory. The making and the marketing of female sex hormones fitted nicely into already existing institutional structures formed earlier in the century. In the process of making female sex hormones into chemical substances, laboratory scientists were able to create networks with gynecologists and pharmaceutical companies prepared to provide them with the required research materials. In the transformation of sex hormones into drugs, we saw a further extension of these networks from the laboratory and the pharmaceutical industry to other medical professions, and to groups beyond the laboratory and the clinic. With respect to female sex hormones, Organon was quite successful in enrolling the relevant groups to promote new types of drugs to a wide variety of audiences, sponsors and consumers, including general practitioners, psychiatrists, neurologists, medical health institutions, women's clinics, factory boards of directors and insurance companies. In the marketing of female sex hormones, the number of indications for which sex hormones were tested increased simultaneously with the involvement of more groups, in a process by which female sex hormones were made into drugs applicable for a wide variety of diseases in women.

What is important here is that some networks are easier to create than others. Negotiations to establish networks do take place in "a highly prestructured reality in which earlier choices delineate the space of further choices" (Berg 1992: 2). In the case of female sex hormones, laboratory scientists and pharmaceutical companies did not have to start from scratch. They could rely on an already organized medical practice that could easily be transformed into an organized market for their products. The gynecological clinic functioned as a powerful institutional context that provided an available and established clientele with a broad range of diseases that could be treated with hormones.

Knowledge claims about male sex hormones were more difficult to link with relevant groups outside the laboratory. The production as well as the marketing of male sex hormones was rather constrained by the lack of an institutional context comparable with the gynecological clinic: men's clinics specializing in the study of the male reproductive system did not exist in the 1920s. The production of male sex hormones was rather problematic because it was hard for laboratory scientists to gain access to the required raw materials. The marketing of male sex hormones remained confined to a smaller number of groups, thus lowering the number of indications that became included in the drug profile of male sex hormones. Although there existed a potential audience for the promotion of male sex hormones, this audience was not embedded in any organized market or resource network. These differences in institutional context had a major impact on the marketing of sex hormones. Because the promotion of female sex hormones could easily be linked to the interests of a well-established profession, female sex hormones developed into drugs that were prescribed for a far wider array of medical indications than male sex hormones.

In the case of sex endocrinology, successes and failures in creating networks were highly dependent on the fact that there existed a medical specialty for the reproductive functions of the female body, and not for the male body. It was this asymmetry in organizational structure that made the female body into the central focus of the hormonal enterprise. Sex endocrinologists depended on these organizational structures to provide them with the necessary tools and materials. These differences in institutionalization between the female and the male body are a very crucial factor in shaping the extent to which knowledge claims can be made into universal facts. The institutionalization of practices concerning the female body in a medical specialty transforms the female body into an easily accessible supplier of research materials, a convenient guinea-pig for tests and an organized audience for the products of science. These established practices facilitated a situation in which the hormonally constructed female body concept acquired its appearance as a universal, natural phenomenon.

The tension between universality and locality

As I have indicated, the transformation of scientific body concepts into natural phenomena requires a second activity: the concealment of contexts. *Beyond the Natural Body* shows that the decontextualized status of scientific knowledge is the result of specific scientific activities. I have described how knowledge claims about sex hormones acquired the status of context-independent facts and artefacts because they became materialized in chemical compounds that could exist independently of the laboratory conditions that shaped them. The history of sex hormones exemplifies how scientists turn observations into materials in which contexts gradually disappear, materials which are subsequently claimed to enjoy an a priori natural existence.

Female sex hormones, for example, have taken on a variety of different forms, showing an increasing degree of context-independency:

1 observations of specific disorders in patients following surgical removal of the ovaries in a gynecological clinic in Vienna
2 preparations of gonads extracted and purified in Laqueur's laboratory in Amsterdam
3 crystals in a bottle on laboratory shelves, carrying an Organon label with a chemical formula
4 pills in a plastic strip provided by health care professionals.

Laboratory experiments have played a major role in this decontextualization of knowledge claims. Scientists used experiments to transform the concept of sex hormones into standardized substances with precisely defined qualities that then became accepted as such by the international scientific community and the industrial world. Subsequently, clinical testing procedures have made these standardized substances available as specific drugs and eventually the pill. Local laboratory practices thus became decontextualized by developing instruments, techniques and standards robust enough to survive outside the laboratory.

However, scientists are not always successful in decontextualizing knowledge claims. There exists a basic tension between scientists' striving for universal, decontextualized knowledge and the notion that science is shaped in its local contexts,[2] a tension with severe practical consequences particularly with respect to the development of (contraceptive) technologies. The decontextualization strategy suggests that technologies can be made to work everywhere, but this is not always so. Scientific artefacts require a specific context in which they can work, one similar to the context from which they arise. If this context is not available, scientists have to create it. Or to use Latour's metaphor of railroads again: scientists first have to construct railroads before the locomotives can move in the envisioned direction. The problem is that for contraceptive technologies such as the pill, the railroads are chiefly constructed in the western industrialized world. Most contraceptive technologies are made in industrialized countries and therefore bear the fingerprints of western producers, including locally and culturally specific ideas of how ideal contraceptives should look like. Every technology contains, so to say, a configured user.[3] Consequently, technologies cannot simply be transported elsewhere.

The case of the contraceptive pill illustrates the complications that emerge if western technologies are introduced into developing countries. Although pill researchers claimed that the pill was a universal, context-independent contraceptive, it nevertheless contained a specific user: a woman, disciplined enough to take medication regularly, who is used to gynecological examinations and regular visits to the physician, and who does not have to hide contraception from her partner. It goes without saying that this portrait of the ideal pill user is highly culturally specific (with varieties even within one culture). This user is more likely to be found in western industrialized countries with well-developed health care systems. From this perspective it can be understood that the pill has not found a universal acceptance. Actually, the user-specificity of the envisioned universal contraceptive pill was already manifest during the clinical testing in Puerto Rico. The early trials witnessed a high percentage of drop-outs. I have described how disciplining women to the conditions of the tests was not always successful. Many women did not participate in the gynecological examinations or simply quit the program because they preferred other contraceptive methods, particularly sterilization. The Puerto Rican trials provided the pill researchers with information indicating that the pill did not meet with universal acceptance. These test conditions were, of course, a much heavier burden than the conditions of using the pill after it had been approved by the FDA. Two conditions remained, however, the same: frequent visits to a physician (the pill was available only on prescription) and regular gynecological examinations (women using the pill had to take regular gynecological examinations, including blood-pressure tests and vaginal smears to check for adverse health effects).[4]

The making of the pill into a successful contraceptive technology thus required a specific context, a context in which

1 there exists an easily accessible, well-developed health care infrastructure
2 people are accustomed to taking prescribed drugs (many developing countries mainly use "over the counter" drugs, which people can buy in shops)
3 women are used to regular medical controls
4 women and men are free to negotiate the use of contraceptives.

The pill could be made into a universal contraceptive only if its producers put great effort into mobilizing and disciplining people and institutions to meet the specific requirements of the new technology. Needless to say, many of the required transformations were beyond the power of the inventors of the pill. The sad conclusion therefore is that, although new contraceptive technologies such as the pill are often tested in Third World countries, the local needs of its potential users are rarely taken into account. During the tests the technologies are more or less successful because scientists make the contexts fit the demands of the testing, for example by enrolling trained medical staff and by selecting trial participants who may be made into ideal test subjects but who are not necessarily representative of the whole population. It is by creating such controlled settings that scientists are able to make the technology work. These controlled settings, however, no longer exist when the trials are over and the technologies are put on the market.

This situation often leads to health risks among the users of the new technologies. Since the 1980s, feminist health organizations seeking safe and reliable contraceptives have reported women's complaints about serious side-effects while using contraceptives such as implants and inject-ables, particularly in developing countries (Anonymous 1985; Mintzes 1992: Ward 1986). Many of these adverse health effects seem to be related to insufficient medical follow-up. These contraceptive technologies all require a health care infrastructure that can provide medical controls for their administration and removal.[5] In many Third World countries, such an infrastructure simply does not exist, particularly in rural areas. To avoid potential health risks, women's health advocates campaign for the development of contraceptives that require less dependency and inter-action with health care providers. They prefer the so-called user-controlled technologies and stress that users' views should be taken into account in assessing acceptability (Bruce 1987; Pollock1984).[6] Scientists in the field of reproductive technology acknowledge the problems with the dif-fusion of new contraceptive technologies and introduced so-called "intro-ductory trials" in the 1980s. These trials were conducted to assess the acceptability of new contraceptives in different social and cultural settings (Hardon and Claudio-Estrada 1991: 12).[7]

These developments exemplify my point that scientific artefacts are not in themselves universal and context-independent. They have to be made into universal technologies by a whole variety of different activities. The introduction of contraceptive technologies shows that science is not always successful in its striving for universal, context-independent knowledge.

THE TRANSFORMATIVE POWER OF SEX HORMONES

What intrigued me most in writing this archeology of sex hormones is the very complex and multileveled impact of the hormonally constructed body concept on our understanding and treatment of the body. The story of hormones exemplifies the transformative power of science and technology. Or to quote Giddens: "Knowledge does not simply render the body more transparent, but alters its nature, spinning it off in novel directions" (Giddens 1990: 153). The interpretation of the body in terms of sex hormones contributed to its transformation, ranging from changes in the very words we use to express our bodily experiences to changes in medical practices and power relations.

The chemical model of sex and the body

The most revolutionary change generated by sex endocrinology is the introduction of a chemical model of sex and the body. I have described how sex endocrinologists introduced the concept of sex hormones as chemical messengers of masculinity and femininity. With the introduction of the concept of sex hormones, sex became attached to chemical sub-stances. The hormonal model of the body is thus basically a chemical model. That scientists at the time were aware of this transformation is exemplified in *The Male Sex Hormone*, a book published in the early 1940s in which the American author describes the role of male hormones in sexual differentiation in terms of "Manhood is chemical" (Kruif undated: 2). The introduction of this chemical model had major consequences for the conceptualization of sex and the body.

First, the very act of attaching sex to chemical substances implies that sex is an entity that can exist apart from any fixed location in the body. If sex is a chemical agent transported by the blood, it can wander around through the whole body. This model meant a crucial change in the conceptualization of sex and the body, both with respect to cultural notions and conceptualizations of preceding disciplines. Prior to the emergence of sex endocrinology, scientists, particularly anatomists, used to locate the "essence" of sex in one specific organ. Femininity was located first in the uterus and later in the ovaries. All through the history of the biomedical sciences, masculinity was primarily located in the testes. Sex endocrinology now had a twofold impact. This new field of the biomedical sciences reinforced, and at the same time challenged, the earlier conceptualization of sex. The introduction of sex hormones as chemical substances secreted by the gonads initially reinforced the cultural notion that the gonads were the seats of masculinity and femininity. Sex endocrinology focused, however, not on the gonads as such, but on their secretions: the chemical substances. In this manner, sex endocrinology transcended the anatomical model of sex and the body in which sex is located in one specific organ. The chemical model enabled scientists to distract attention away from the gonads as the organs where sex is located. Sex endocrinologists included the hypophysis in the hormonal model of the body, thus extending the "essence" of sex from the gonads to the brain. In the hormonal model, sex is no longer located in one specific organ, but develops in a complex feedback system between the gonads and the brain. This conceptualization of sex and the body meant a break with the cultural notion that masculinity and femininity are solely located in the gonads.[8] It also meant a break with the anatomical model of sex and the body.

Second, the introduction of the chemical model led to a shift away from a primarily descriptive approach and toward an experimental approach. While anatomists focused on identifying which organ is the seat of femininity or masculinity, sex endocrinologists looked for the causal mechanisms that control sexual differentiation. Sex endocrinology is basically an experimental science. Locating the "essence" of sex in chemical substances implies that sex is an entity that can be identified and isolated from the organism. Locating sex in chemicals means that there can be too much or too little of these substances in the organism. Sex thus becomes an entity that can be measured, quantified and manipulated with laboratory techniques. Consequently, sex endocrinology became a science that actively intervenes in the lives of women and men, introducing diagnostic and intervention techniques that have profoundly shaped medical practice.

Finally, a chemical model of sex and the body makes it possible to abandon a rigorous dualistic notion of sex, a notion characteristic of cultural ideas of sex differences and of the anatomical model of sex. If one locates the "essence" of sex in specific sex organs such as the gonads, masculinity and femininity can be conceptualized in terms of mutually exclusive entities. In this model, male bodies are simply male, and female bodies simply female. Attaching sex to chemicals rather than organs means that sex becomes an entity with multidirectional capacities. Sex endocrinologists introduced a quantitative model of sex differences, in which all organisms can have feminine as well as masculine characteristics. The original assumption that each sex could be recognized by its own sex hormone was gradually replaced by a model in which male and female sex hormones are present in both sexes. Yet sex endocrinologists did not take the real challenge that their model provided, namely to abandon the dualistic notion that there exist only two sexes. From a standpoint of gender classifications, their revolutionary findings did not mean the end of the two-sexes model. Based on the same knowledge, it might have been possible to introduce a classification system of multiple sexes, just as has been suggested by Anne Fausto-Sterling (1993). In "Five Sexes: Why Male and Female are not Enough", Fausto-Sterling suggested that "biologically speaking, there are many gradations running from female to male; and depending on how one calls the shots, one can argue that along that spectrum lie at least five sexes – and perhaps even more" (Fausto-Sterling 1993: 21). The new science of sex endocrinology, however, decided to adhere to the traditional gender classification system.[9]

Cyclicity versus stability

The chemical model of sex was a rather radical model because it reduced the differences between the sexes to one hydroxyl group: men and women differ only in the relative amounts of their sex hormones. This does not mean that sex endocrinology did not emphasize differences between the female and the male body. In addition to the chemical model, sex endocrinology also provided a model in which sex differences came to be conceptualized in terms of the rhythm of hormone production. Biologists and gynecologists specified the quantitative theory of sex differences in terms of the notion that the male and the female body differ from each other with respect to their hormone regulation. Gynecologists used the hormonal blood test to specify the nature of hormone regulation in the female and the male body. Based on this test, the female body became characterized by its cyclic hormonal regulation and the male body by its stable hormonal regulation. In this biological context, sex differences thus became conceptualized in terms of cyclicity versus stability.

This association of femininity with cyclicity was not entirely new. In the second half of the nineteenth century, psychiatrists became interested in the "periodic madnesses" of their female patients and ascribed these to the cyclic nature of their menstruation. At the turn of the century, the German psychiatrist Krafft-Ebing questioned the "mental integrity" of menstruating women (Baart and Bransen 1986: 8). This association of femininity with cyclicity was thus compatible with notions about femininity that already existed in culture and medical practice. What is new is that sex endocrinologists transformed this notion of cyclicity into a basic model for understanding the specific nature of the physical features of the female body. They linked cyclicity with a chemical substance, regulating the development of a wider variety of functions than just reproductive functions. This extension of the concept of cyclicity is exemplified in the handbook *Female Sex Endocrinology* (1949):

> the complete physical and mental structure of a woman is, just as her reproductive functions, exposed to cyclic stimulation of sex hormones. This is not only manifest in the cyclic changes in the endometrium, but also in fluctuations in temperament, changes in breast size, heart beat, and so on.
>
> (Binsberg 1949: 1)

Sex endocrinologists thus redefined the meanings assigned to femininity, emphasizing cyclicity as the key concept for understanding the female body.[10]

In this case, we see how sex endocrinology incorporates cultural norms and – at the same time – actively reshapes these ideas. A similar pattern can be distinguished in the manner in which sex endocrinology conceptualized the female body in terms of its reproductive functions. In the hormone model, the female body became increasingly defined as a reproductive entity. The image of the female body as primarily a reproductive body has a long history manifest in many cultures. Foucault described how in the late eighteenth and early nineteenth centuries scientists incorporated this cultural notion into the medical sciences. In this period, medical scientists increasingly defined the female body as an object of sexuality and reproduction (Foucault 1984: 104, 115, 119). Sex endocrinologists integrated the notion of the female body as a reproductive body into the hormonal model, but not without thoroughly changing it. They introduced highly technical tools to investigate the female reproductive functions to an extent that was not possible before. Sex endocrinologists shaped medical practice most profoundly, because they provided the medical profession with tools to intervene in features that had been considered inaccessible prior to the hormonal era. The introduction of diagnostic tests and drugs enabled the medical profession to intervene in the menstrual cycle and the menopause, thus bringing the "natural" features of reproduction and aging into the domain of medical intervention.

Living in the material world

Beyond the Natural Body shows that the power to control sex and the body is embodied not only in scientific theory, but also in materialities. This is why I suggested that it is crucial for feminist studies of science to take into account this materiality of the scientific enterprise. The suggestion that science is primarily texts and theories seriously fails to take into account the strongest tools that scientists have at hand to transform and sexualize the world we live in: the creation of material products. A focus on the materiality of science shows how the construction of meanings and practices of sex and the body is not restricted to the domain of theories and semiotics.

In the first place, sex endocrinology produced new diagnostic techniques. The use of tests introduced for measuring hormones in animals did not remain restricted to the laboratory. Clinicians, particularly gynecologists, transferred the laboratory tests to the clinic as tools for the diagnosis of hormonal deficiences. Laboratory scientists introduced three types of tests: the sex hormone blood test (one to estimate male sex hormones, one to estimate female sex hormones), the pregnancy test and the vaginal smear test. Clinicians used the sex hormone blood test to measure the sex of homosexual men and to classify women into hormonal types. The female sex hormone blood test was also used for the diagnosis of menstrual disorders and pregnancy. The pregnancy test became widely used as the first laboratory test for the early diagnosis of pregnancy. The introduction of the vaginal smear test provided gynecologists and physicians with a powerful new diagnostic tool to investigate their female patients. They have used this test for the diagnosis of menstrual disorders, and more recently for the diagnosis of cancer. The introduction of this test profoundly shaped the medical treatment of the female body, extending medical intervention techniques from the uterus and the ovaries to the vagina.

In addition to the introduction of diagnostic techniques, sex endocrinology provided the medical profession with a new class of drugs that were developed to cure a newly constructed category of diseases: hormone deficiency diseases. Sex endocrinologists defined low levels of hormones as deficiencies. In this manner, they transformed the hormonal model of sex into a model of disorders and pathologies. The concept of hormonal deficiency disease implies that this category of diseases can be treated with the administration of hormones to make up for the lack of these substances. I described how this hormonal model of diseases became integrated into medical practice. The introduction of hormones as drugs had a major impact on medical practice, particularly on women, since it was the female body that became increasingly subjected to medical intervention. The specification of the hormone model of the female body as cyclic in nature further facilitated the process of classifying women's diseases in terms of deficiencies that could be treated with hormones. The introduction of the pill, last but not least, revolutionalized sexual experiences by providing a means to separate sexuality from reproduction.

The introduction of the concept of sex hormones not only changed the medical treatment of the human body, but also redefined the existing social configurations structuring medical practice. The story about hormones thus becomes a story about power and medicine. The field of sex endocrinology generated a set of power relations that did not exist prior to its emergence. What changed in this period was the question of who was entitled to claim authoritative knowledge about the female body. The introduction of the hormonal model increased the medical authority of gynecologists over disorders traditionally belonging to other medical professions, such as psychiatry. The hormonal model thus enabled gynecologists to draw the female body more and more deeply into the gynecological clinic. Gynecologists, however, had to share their increased medical authority with another professional group: the laboratory scientists. With the introduction of the concept of sex hormones, scientists explicitly linked women's diseases with laboratory practice. Laboratory scientists entered a field until then relatively untouched by laboratory science. Before the turn of the century, the study of women's diseases, traditionally ascribed to dysfunction of the ovaries, was the exclusive field of gynecologists. In the decades to follow, research on the ovaries shifted from the clinic to the laboratory. Laboratory scientists succeeded in becoming experts on disorders in the ovaries and female reproduction. In this manner, laboratory scientists gained a new realm of influence, claiming authoritative knowledge over a subject previously allocated to gynecologists. The gynecologists thus lost their position as the sole experts on women's diseases and reproduction.

This story of hormones is a story of multiple and mobile power relations, very similar to Foucault's accounts of power (Foucault 1975; 1976). Here power is not a fixed, homogeneous thing, located in one specific place or institution, neither is it possessed by one specific actor. My account of the history of sex hormones shows the dynamic, capillary power of a science which linked cultural assumptions, concepts, ovaries, urine, diagnostic tests, lab equipment, marketing strategies, clinical trials, population policies and bodies, thus transforming the world we live in. *Beyond the Natural Body* shows the enormous transformative power of biomedicine: a world with hormones looks quite different from a world without them. Sex hormones shaped our understanding of sex and the body, they changed the medical treatment of our bodies, they constituted a new specialty in the biomedical sciences, they thoroughly changed the cultural and material authority of the laboratory and the clinic, and last but not least, sex hormones redefined the relationship of women to reproduction.

THE MIXED BLESSINGS OF SEX HORMONES

In this epilogue it is time to reflect on what sex hormones have brought us. Clearly, hormones have changed our world. The quest for sex hormones exemplifies the dreams of modernity. The promises of the new science of sex endocrinology mirror the modernist claim that "a progressive growth of scientific knowledge will uncover the natural order of things, making possible the construction of techologies through which control might be exercised over the course of the development of events" (Smart 1992: 56). In this Enlightenment tradition, science and technology are considered as intrinsically progressive and beneficial. The role of science and technology in our society is perceived as improving the "human" condition.

The quest for sex hormones was firmly rooted in this belief of science as progress. Since its early years, the science of sex hormones promised to provide a technological fix for many problems, particularly "women's problems." Robert Frank's *The Female Sex Hormone* very vividly illustrates this modernist tradition when the author promises his readers that female sex hormones are "bound to relieve many of the ills from which women suffer" (Frank 1929: Introduction). The intriguing question is: has Frank's dream come true? My book would have a happy end, providing the answer is a straightforward yes. Unfortunately, but not unexpectedly, the answer is not that easy. The introduction of the hormonally constructed body concept has led to a situation in which "control can be exercised across the life course from menstruation through menopause" (Clarke 1990a). So far, we may be inclined to conclude that Robert Frank was right and very much ahead of his time. We may question, however, whether and to what extent sex hormones are an adequate solution for "women's problems." Undoubtly, many women will emphasize the benefits of hormone therapy. Yet it is the very idea of control and the awareness of (potential) health hazards that turned the dream of hormones as problem solvers into a reality of growing ambivalence and severe criticism. Two examples of the use of sex hormones, the pill and hormone replacement therapy, clearly illustrate the two faces of the hormonal revolution.

The story of the pill is a story about liberation and control. On the one hand the pill is "except for the word 'no' the most effective and convenient contraceptive ever devised," a technology that contributed to the increasing liberation of women (Seaman and Seaman 1977: 95). On the other hand it is a story about Western science ignoring the local needs of specific users, particularly the communities on the Caribbean islands and other Third World countries. The "one size fits all"[11] approach to making contraceptives such as the pill does not acknowledge diversities among women. I have argued that these universal tendencies are highly problematic because they cause serious health risks. Moreover, in the domain of population policy, the pill is not unproblematic because it serves as a tool in the pursuit of a technological fix for problems which ultimately are political, economic, cultural and moral in kind.

A similar story can be told for the use of sex hormones for the treatment of menopausal symptoms. Since the 1960s hormone replacement therapy for menopausal women has become very popular, particularly in the United States, where the sales of estrogen preparations have quadrupled. Today these drugs are even one of the top five prescription drugs (Greer 1991: 185). Again, the use of hormones has two faces. It promises a relief of many negative bodily experiences during aging. Many women consider hormone replacement therapy as an efficient therapy and as an acknowledgement of their problems by the medical profession. The other face is more gloomy. It shows the many controversies that have accompanied the introduction of hormone replacement therapy. There are the recurring debates about risks of cancer and other serious side-effects. There is the criticism on the reductionist view on menopause: hormonal explanations of menopause reduce the complexity of aging to a disease entity. (Greer 1991; Seaman and Seaman 1977).

In summary, sex hormones may best be portrayed as a mixed blessing. The implication of my remarks is not a cultural or technological pessimism but rather that we need to understand science and technology with all its tensions and ambiguities. My argument throughout this book has been that bodies and technologies are not unequivocally determined by nature. Medical technologies do not necessarily have to be the way they actually are. Who knows what might have happened to the hormonally constructed body concept if there had existed an andrological clinic, rather than a gynecological clinic? Imagine what might have happened in a world with different cultural and moral attitudes towards gender and responsibilities for family planning and childcare. It is not beyond imagination that we would have ended up with a male contraceptive pill, a medical treatment of male menopause and a classification system of multiple sexes. Alas, we will never know whether this really would have happened. We know, however, one thing for sure: science and technology can take many shapes. A critical deconstruction of the processes that shape science, technology and bodies might help us to envisage technologies that have a chance of survival.

Notes

1 INTRODUCTION

1 For a more comprehensive analysis of the attitudes of early feminism toward biology, see Birke (1986: 1–13).

2 Oakley (1972). The use of the concept of gender in scientific discourse is not restricted to the feminist research of the 1970s, but dates from the 1930s. Psychologists introduced this category to study masculine and feminine psychological and behavioral characteristics, because they considered physiological differences to be inadequate markers of the attributes of men and women. The psychologists Lewis Terman and Catherine Cox Miles developed techniques to identify and measure the "psychological gender attributes" of women and men that became the prototype for research on femininity and masculinity for over three decades in psychological research: see Lewin (1984); Shaver and Hendrick (1987: 45).

3 For a more detailed analysis of these strategies in feminist research, see Mol (1988).

4 There is one major exception: in *The Woman in the Body*, Emily Martin (1987) includes a deconstruction of medical views of the reproductive functions of the female body.

5 Bleier (1984; 1986); Hubbard (1981); Hubbard *et al.* (1982); Keller (1982; 1984); Longino (1990); Longino and Doell (1983). In contrast to feminist sociologists, feminist biologists considered the body as relevant for the feminist research agenda. Actually, feminist biologists have adopted this position from the very beginning of the debate about sex and gender. My account of the history of feminist studies should therefore not be read as a story of continuity and progress. There have been, and still are, many different positions in the debate about sex, gender and the body.

6 There is, of course, the important question of the extent to which women adopt biomedical knowledge in understanding of their bodies. In *Woman Beneath the Skin: A Doctor's Patients in Eighteenth-century Germany*, Barbara Duden argues that body perception has two very different histories dealing with two different traditions: the tradition of the oral culture and the written medical tradition. Duden suggests that the woman's body should be understood in terms of "a fragile synthesis" of these two traditions (Duden 1991c: 35, 182). In *The Woman in the Body*, Emily Martin concludes that all women are affected in one way or another by biomedical views of physical life events such as menstruation, menopause and childbirth. She showed important differences in the extent to which women accept or resist this knowledge. Middle-class women in the USA (black or white) readily inclined toward the medical view of their bodies, explaining reproductive processes in terms of

"internal organs, structures, and functions" (Martin 1987: 105). Working-class women, on the other hand, seem to share an absolute resistance to this medical view, and explain their bodies in terms of what a woman sees or feels or the significance it has in her life (Martin 1987: 109).

7 See, among other, Bijker and Law (1992); Bijker *et al.* (1987); Gilbert and Mulkay (1984a); Latour (1987); Latour and Woolgar (1979).

8 See for example Bell (1987); Birke (1986); Bleier (1984; 1986); Clarke (1990a); Fausto-Sterling (1985); Haraway (1981; 1989b); Honegger (1991); Hubbard (1981); Hubbard *et al.* (1982); Jacobus *et al.* (1990); Jordanova (1980; 1989); Laqueur (1990); Longino (1990); Longino and Doell (1983); Mol (1988); Sayers (1982); Schiebinger (1986; 1989); Wijngaard (1991a; 1991b).

9 In the context of this book I discuss only the feminist literature. The social shaping of medicine and the body is also described by "mainstream" historians, anthropologists and sociologists: see among others Feher *et al.* (1989).

10 Ludmilla Jordonova gave another striking example in her analysis of the representation of the female and the male body in the wax models used for making anatomical drawings in the biomedical sciences in France and Britain in the eighteenth and nineteenth centuries. She described how these wax models depict male figures as active agents and females as the passive objects of sexual desire. The female figures, or "Venuses," lie on the velvet or silk cushions, whereas male figures are usually upright, and often in positions of motion, thus reflecting the cultural stereotypes of the active male and the passive female (Jordanova 1980: 54).

11 This shift seems to have been caused by epistemological and socio-political changes rather than by scientific progress. In *Making Sex*, Thomas Laqueur described this shift in the context of changes in the political climate. The French Revolution and new liberal claims in the seventeenth century led to new ideals about the social relationships between men and women, in which the complementarity between the sexes was emphasized. This theory of com-plementarity "taught that men and women are not physical and moral equals but complementary opposites." Women now became viewed as "fundamentally different from, and thus incomparable to, men" (T. Laqueur 1990: 32, 216, 217). The theory of sexual complementarity was meant to keep women out of competition with men, designing separate spheres for men and women. In this theory, which came to be known as the "doctrine of the two spheres," the sexes were expected to complement, rather than compete with, each other.

   The shift from studying similarities to differences was not caused by new scientific findings; on the contrary, Laqueur described how scientific literature provided many new discoveries which could have strengthened the one-sex model. The new field of embryology, for instance, claimed that reproductive organs "begin from one and the same embryonic structure," offering support to the earlier belief in the similarity between male and female reproductive systems (T. Laqueur 1990: 169). However, Laqueur does not present a simple causal model for scientific and political changes: "these social and political changes are not, in themselves, explanations for the reinterpretation of bodies ... none of these things caused the making of a new sex body. Instead, the remaking of the body is itself intrinsic to each of these developments" (T. Laqueur 1990: 11).

12 See Briscoe (1978); Fausto-Sterling (1985); Fried (1982); Messent (1976); Money and Ehrhardt (1972); Rogers (1976).

13 The literature of social studies of science provides two different perspectives within the network approach: the actor-network model and the social network model. The (predominantly French) actor-network theorists depict scientific knowledge as a result of "heterogeneous networks," that is networks of people,

machines, organizations and knowledge. These theorists make no analytical distinctions between human and non-human actors. Material elements, such as electrons and catalysts, are portrayed as actors in their own right. In contrast to the actor-network theorists, the Anglo-Saxon social network theorists restrict the notion of networks to human actors. These studies describe how the structural characteristics of interrelations between people influence human action. Social network theorists suggest that the freedom of scientists to realize their interests is to a large extent shaped by their positions in the network and their relations with other groups in the network. One of the major representatives of the social network theorists is Ronald Burt (1982), who develops mathematical models to capture the patterns of relations in social networks and uses these models to describe the social structures of two systems of actors: large American manufacturing concerns and elite experts in sociological methodology. In this study, I adopt the theoretical premises of the social network approach, but will not develop any mathematical models. For a further description of this strand of network analysis, see also Burt and Minor (1983); Knoke and Kuklinsky (1982). Ever since its introduction, the notion of "networks" has been given many different meanings in a variety of contexts; for a detailed description of the different perspectives, see Blauwhof et al. (1990).

14 Historians and sociologists of the biomedical sciences emphasize that the development of the biomedical sciences is a multidisciplinary endeavor, embodying not only the dynamics of the biological and chemical sciences, but also the dynamics of medical practice and industrial corporations (Amsterdamska 1987; Bell 1986; Blume 1992). From this perspective, hormones are the embodiment of complex historical and sociological processes involving interactions between biological and chemical laboratories, clinics, and pharmaceutical companies. In this study I distinguish laboratory scientists and clinicians, not because clinicians did not do any laboratory research, but merely to emphasize the different contexts in which research on sex hormones took place. I use the term "laboratory scientists" for those researchers who, as against clinicians, performed research unconnected with any clinical practice.

15 In the early decades of the eighteenth century, when the medical sciences were dominated by the theory of the mixture of humors, the idea of impure blood was framed in terms of a "foul mixture of humors." In the late nineteenth century, when the chemical approach became more dominant, syphilis was described in terms of "the changed chemistry of the blood." Finally, with the emergence of bacteriology in the early decades of the twentieth century, the concept of syphilis assumed its current form, in which the prescientific idea of impure blood became framed in terms of biological causal agents: bacteria.

16 Fleck introduced the concept of "thought styles" to address differences in styles between "thought collectives." Although Fleck did not restrict this concept to scientific disciplines, he did write about differences in thought styles between disciplines, comparing physicists with biologists (Fleck 1979: 64, 92, 108).

17 I draw specifically on the conceptual work of Michel Foucault, who first introduced the concepts of archeology and discourse in the history and philosophy of the (biomedical) sciences. The material conditions of knowledge production are very central in Foucault's work. In this choice, he was inspired by the French philosopher Canguilhem, who emphasized the intertwining of concepts and techniques: see Canguilhem (1977); Foucault (1975; 1976); Mol and Lieshout (1989). My approach is different from Foucault's approach in

the sense that I focus more exclusively on what happens in the laboratory and in the content of science and technology.

18 In *Making Sex*, Laqueur does not focus on the materiality of knowledge production, although his historical sources, at least on one occasion, pointed very clearly in this direction. In his analysis of early anatomical practices, he describes how in the fifteenth- and sixteenth-century anatomy books the body being dissected is male. Laqueur only occasionally mentions that this might be due to "the availability of material rather than sexual politics." To gain access to corpses, anatomists depended on executions, and since more men than women were executed, female corpses were rather scarce material (T. Laqueur 1990: 74).

19 The issue of practices, in a broader sense, has been addressed by feminist scholars in the literary and cultural sciences. Alcoff (1988) emphasizes the need for feminists to devote more attention to practices in order to avoid depicting the world as consisting merely of texts and constructions. Lauretis (1984) stresses that sex differences are constructed not only in language: habits and practices are crucial in the construction of meanings.

20 Studies of the role of experimental and testing practices include Franklin (1986); Galison (1987); Gilbert and Mulkay (1984b); Gooding *et al.* (1989); Hacking (1986); Pinch (1993); Shapin and Schaffer (1985). Studies giving detailed accounts of laboratory life include Collins (1975); Collins and Pinch (1982); Knorr-Cetina (1981a); Latour and Woolgar (1979); Lynch (1985); Travis (1981).

21 The scope of the scientific literature analyzed is limited to basic and clinical research on sex hormones undertaken by researchers in biology, chemistry and medicine, excluding agricultural scientists. The empirical data are derived from a variety of sources. The analysis of the international field of sex endocrinology (Chapters 2, 3 and 6) is based on publications from American, British and German biomedical and chemical journals published between 1920 and 1940 (Chapters 2 and 3) and in the late 1950s and early 1960s (Chapter 6); historical reviews of these periods; reports of the International Conferences on Standardization of Sex Hormones held in London in 1932, 1935 and 1938; and the *Quarterly Cumulative Index Medicus* from 1927 to 1938. The analysis of Dutch sex endocrinology is based on two major Dutch journals, *The Dutch Journal of Medicine (Nederlands Tijdschrift voor Geneeskunde)*, 1920–1940, and *The Hormone (Het Hormoon)*, 1923–1940; on the Organon Archives; particularly the correspondence of Ernst Laqueur with Organon employees, 1923–1940; and on personal interviews with (the now late) Prof. Dr. Marius Tausk, the medical director of Organon in the 1920s and 1930s, and with Dr. Ina Uyldert, a biologist who has worked since the 1920s at the Pharmaco-Therapeutic Laboratory of the University of Amsterdam.

2 THE BIRTH OF SEX HORMONES

1 There were differences between Europe and the United States in respect of the biological specialties involved in early hormone research. In Europe, physiologists were the major laboratory scientists of the first generation of sex endocrinologists. In the USA many of the major laboratory scientists were zoologists and anatomists: see Clarke (1985). But see Long (1987) for a different view of disciplines and sex endocrinology in the American context. Long described how "during the interwar period, the new field of endocrinology was closely associated with the older discipline of physiology" (Long 1987: 263).

2 This shift of emphasis can be traced, at least in part, to the laboratory scientists' tendency to move away from therapeutic concerns toward the more reductionist approach of the new professional scientist (Long Hall 1976).

3 For an extensive description of early ideas of the testes, see Hamilton (1986: 12–15).

4 For a description of the work of Brown-Séquard, see Borell (1976b: 235); Corner (1965: 5).

5 For a description of the introduction of the theory of internal secretions, see Borell (1976a; 1976b).

6 Early descriptions of the uterus can be traced back to antiquity in Sumerian, Egyptian, Hebrew, Greek and Roman sources. The first known description of the ovary as an anatomic unit goes back to about 300 BC. Vesalius, often portrayed as the "Father of Modern Anatomy," is mostly thought to have been the first anatomist to have described the ovarian follicles. In 1672, Regnier de Graaf first introduced the concept of the ovary as the producer of eggs. All early scholars studying the ovary described the anatomic unit as "the female testicle": see Gruhn and Kazer (1989: 3–16).

7 The fact that European gynecologists (in particular Viennese gynecologists) were the first to recognize the relevence of the theory of internal secretions to the ovaries is described in Borell (1985: 13).

8 In the period under study, this new field in the life sciences was known as sex endocrinology. The term "reproductive endocrinology," by which this field is now known, originates from a later period. Given this historical background, I shall use the term "sex endocrinology."

9 Adele Clarke (1985) argues that this taboo subsequently delayed the development of reproductive science: see Aberle and Corner (1953) on the role of taboo in sex research.

10 The role of a chromosomal factor in sex determination was first mentioned by the American zoologist Clarence I. McClung. In 1902 McClung published his report on sex determination in the *Biological Bulletin*, in which he described the structures that would eventually become known as the sex chromosomes: see Money (1980: 2).

11 Long Hall (1975: 86–87). These early studies of what has now become known as the prenatal effects of hormones on the sexual development of the embryo preluded a new line of inquiry that remained largely unexplored till the early 1950s. In that period French embryologists took up this line of inquiry, exploring the role of sex hormones in the sexual differentiation of the genital tract of the embryo. In the late 1950s, American biologists extended this research to the sexual differentiation of the brain. In 1959 William Young, a professor in the Department of Anatomy of the University of Kansas, and his colleagues Phoenix, Goy and Gerall introduced a theory on the prenatal effects of hormones on brain tissues mediating mating behavior. The introduction of this "organization" theory preluded the emergence of neuro-endocrinology as a new field in the life sciences in the 1960s. For an extensive reconstruction of the history of this line of inquiry, see Wijngaard (1991b). In contrast to this later development, in which endocrinologists focussed particularly on the role of sex hormones in producing changes in the brain tissues of the embryo (now known as organizational effects), the early sex endocrinologists focussed primarily on the role of sex hormones in the adult organism (now known as activational effects).

12 For a further description of the controversy about sex determination, see Long Hall (1975).

13 Steinach had developed this antagonistic hypothesis to explain his experiences with unsuccessful gonad transplantations. In a series of publications from 1910

to 1920 he reported his observations on antagonism between the ovaries and the testes when young male and female rats and guinea-pigs were implanted with gonads of the other sex. Gonad grafts survived in hosts of the other sex only when the gonads were removed. Later in the 1920s Steinach extended his conceptualization and applied it directly to the hormones themselves and not merely to interactions between the gonads. In 1926 he reported an antagonistic influence of female sex hormones upon both the gonad and secondary sexual characteristics of the male. In the same period similar reports were published of what was called an 'antimasculine' activity of sex hormones: see Moore and Price (1932); Steinach (1926).

14 Unfortunately, Fellner's publication could not be traced by the university library system in Amsterdam. Owing to this, I was not able to analyze the original text in order to describe Fellner's motives and interpretations of these experiments.

15 The issue of research materials will be dealt with in more detail in Chapter 4.

16 The impact of Zondek's publication on the field of sex endocrinology can be derived from the *Quarterly Cumulative Index Medicus*. The number of reports published on female sex hormones in male organisms, as registered in this *Index*, increased from nine in 1928 to thirty-five in 1935 and forty-two in 1936, and declined to fifteen in 1937. If we calculate with a delay in the intake of publications by the *Index Medicus* of one year, we see a peak in the number of publications in 1934 and 1935, shortly after Zondek's publication. The peak in publications on male sex hormones in female organisms appeared two years later.

17 Zondek (1934b: 494). Historians of science usually portray Bernhard Zondek as the "discoverer" of the presence of female sex hormones in males. However, as we have seen, Zondek was certainly not the first scientist to report on this. This is a common phenomenon in the history of science. The scientist named as the "discoverer" of a certain finding is not necessarily the only one involved in the issue. In this case, Zondek cannot be seen in isolation from the context of his colleagues, who were all involved in testing the paradigm of sex hormones. Kuhn (1970) described the development of scientific discoveries. According to Kuhn, discoveries cannot be regarded as isolated acts that can be assigned to individual scientists. Instead, Kuhn argues that discoveries should be considered as more extensive episodes in the development of a scientific field in which the adjustment of concepts takes place. It is likely that the attention of historians of science is so exclusively focussed on Zondek because he was the first to publish his observations in a journal for a wider public: *Nature*.

18 In the period from 1927 to 1939, fifty-three articles on the presence of female hormones in male organisms and fourteen articles on the presence of male hormones in female organisms were indexed in the *Quarterly Cumulative Index Medicus*. The number of publications on the function and effects of male sex hormones in the female body indexed in the same period is considerably less than the number of publications on the functions and effects of female sex hormones in the male body (79 and 138 respectively). In the period from 1927 to 1938 the total number of publications on sex hormones indexed in the *Quarterly Cumulative Index Medicus* rose from 95 to 826.

19 In mentioning the presence of female sex hormones in males, I also refer to the presence of male sex hormones in females, in order to avoid a continuous repetition of the same phrase. I shall make a differentiation only if the history on male sex hormones in females diverges from the history of female sex hormones in males. However, at some points this differentiation cannot be

made because the condition of males regarding female sex hormones has been more thoroughly studied than the condition of females.

20 Laqueur's colleague Freud should not, of course, be taken for Sigmund Freud. Although Sigmund Freud did not participate in hormone research, he "postulated something akin to sexual hormones in *Three Essays on the Theory of Sexuality* (1905) well before these hormones were discovered" (Brennan 1992: 140).

21 Authors who reported on female sex hormones causing disease in male bodies, included Beck and Schmitz (1936); Santgiorgi (1937); Toulouse *et al.* (1935). For a critical evaluation of hormonal studies on homosexuality, see Meyer-Bahlburg (1977; 1984).

22 Although this theory was constructed in close cooperation between Carl Moore and Dorothy Price, the theory is generally referred to as Moore's theory of endocrine feedback. According to her personal account of the development of this theory (Price 1975), the original concept was actually developed by Dorothy Price.

23 In this classification Korenchevsky attributed a sexual identity to the hormone itself. This practice of naming was rather common in the 1920s. The literature in this period is scattered with names like "homosexual hormones" (referring to female sex hormones in female organisms) and "heterosexual hormones" (referring to female sex hormones in male organisms). This type of naming was heavily criticized by Alan S. Parkes (1938: 141).

24 It is striking that during the three International Conferences on Standardization of Sex Hormones held in London during the 1930s, the very names of male and female sex hormones were never discussed.

25 The terminological practice in the scientific community in the 1920s and 1930s can be derived from the titles of publications indexed in the *Quarterly Cumulative Index Medicus* in the period from 1927 to 1937. The titles show that the names male and female sex hormones began to be questioned from the beginning of the 1930s. In 1931 the first title appeared with the name "ambosexual hormone" (vol. 9) and in 1933 the first title appeared in which the author referred to the hormone as the "so-called female sex hormone" (vol. 13). The nomenclature for male sex hormones changes after 1936. In that year the first publication appeared with the name "male" hormone (vol. 19). In 1937 the terms "androgens" and "estrogens" were introduced as subject entries. From the moment of introduction, more publications were indexed under the subject entries androgens and estrogens than under the other subject entries (like sex hormones, ovarian hormones and internal secretions of testicles). In a rather short period the names androgens and estrogens were accepted as general terms for sex hormones.

26 See Schiebinger (1986) for a comprehensive analysis of the history of the study of sex since the sixteenth century.

27 Caldwell *et al.* (1934). For a detailed study of the history of pelvimetry, see Hiddinga (1990).

3 THE MEASURING OF SEX HORMONES

1 Many endocrinologists, untrained in the study of animal behavior, were distressed by the variability, or as they saw it, the unreliability of behavioral responses to hormone preparations: see Beach (1981: 335, 337).

2 The uterus test was criticized as a specific bio-assay for female sex hormones because the growth of the uterus could also be affected by means of other substances such as liver extracts: see Dongen (1929).

3 Zondek and Finkelstein (1966: 5). One prominent scientist in the 1920s and 1930s, the American anatomist George W. Corner, even testified in the late 1930s, for the United States Food and Drug Administration in a lawsuit entitled "The United States against four dozen tablets of corpora lutea substance." Corner claimed that the tablets, made from sows' ovaries, contained neither of the ovarian hormones known in the 1930s: see Corner (1965: 6).

4 J. Freud (1936). Even in more recent times, the unitary school seems to be dominating the field of endocrinology. In 1984 the American endocrinologist Richard Whalen advised his colleagues to be more cautious in naming hormones:

> Our scientific language is often misleading. This brief review is intended as a reminder that androgens, oestrogens and other steroid hormones should be considered as merely labels that are used to describe one, often prominent, biological action of these compounds. The caution to be drawn is that none of these agents is entirely specific; all have multiple effects. We should be sensitive to this fact both in our everyday scientific language and in our thoughts about mechanisms of action by which these drugs mediate their effects.

> (Whalen 1984)

5 Prior to the introduction of urine as a research material, scientists used materials that required relatively simple preparatory techniques, such as crushing and filtering methods. The processing of urine demanded more complicated extraction methods, including chemical analytical methods.

6 The behavioral tests had similar disadvantages, being extremely time-consuming. Recording the sexual receptivity of rats involved testing every animal every hour 24 hours per day: see Beach (1981: 335, 337).

7 For a reconstruction of the work of George Papanicolaou, see Clarke (1993).

8 For a detailed historical analysis of Hirschfeld's *Zwischenstufentheorie* and his relations with Steinach, see Schmidt (1984).

9 For a more extended analysis of how the classification of homosexuality became entangled with the classification of gender, see Oudshoorn (1994).

10 This analysis of the *Dutch Journal for Medicine* was made by Ellen Mookhoek as part of the seminar Women's Studies and Medical History, University of Amsterdam, 1991.

11 University laboratories played a major role in setting standards for measurement in many fields of the natural sciences. Simon Schaffer (1990), analyzing the introduction of the Ohm as the international standard of resistance, described how university laboratories established their status as indispensible for setting standards, creating relations of dependencies with industrial companies that are comparable to the field of sex hormones.

4 THE MAKING OF SEX HORMONES

1 In the pharmaceutical industry, animal organs were in fact used in two ways: both as research materials and as raw materials for the production of gonadal preparations. Research in the pharmaceutical industry focussed mainly on investigating the means of extraction of the hormones from natural sources and the means of synthesizing them in order to produce or manufacture them. Research at the Dutch pharmaceutical company Organon also included the performance of bio-assays in order to test the quality of the hormone products. In this chapter I shall not differentiate between research materials and raw materials, because the same materials were used in both contexts.

2 The function of abattoirs in providing the scientists with the required research materials has been discussed by Clarke (1987b: 329–331).

3 Source: Notes of the meetings of the City Council of Amsterdam: Gemeenteblad afd 1 no. 598 Pharmaco-therapeutisch Laboratorium en Gemeenteblad afd 1 no. 760 Pharmaco-therapeutisch Laboratorium.

4 Source: Notes of the extraordinary meeting of guardians: "Buitengewone vergadering van curatoren 22 juni 1931 om twee uur ten stadhuize."

5 Laqueur *et al.* (1927a). Laqueur's American colleague, the biochemist Edward Doisy, also complained about the high cost of sows' ovaries, which in his opinion delayed the isolation of female sex hormones: see Doisy (1972: 701).

6 In the 1930s, the analysis of the hormone content of urine had developed into a general diagnostic method in the clinic. Gynecologists expected that the excretion of hormones in urine indicated an abnormally high quantity of hormones in the female body, which was considered to be the cause of female disorders: see E. Laqueur (1937). However, in the late 1930s, gynecologists suggested that the relationship between illness and the excretion of hormones was not so simple: see Tausk (1938a).

7 Parkes (1985: 125). The activity of ovarian extracts was measured by monitoring the effects of the extract on the cornification of cells in the vagina of the castrated animals. Hormone preparations made from urine had a more pronounced effect on changes in the vaginal cells than preparations made from the ovaries.

8 In the 1920s, Bernhard Zondek worked for some years as an employee of Organon. Organon, as well as Zondek's colleagues, were impressed by Zondek's suggestion that urine was the ideal source for female sex hormones: see Tausk (1978: 30).

9 The practice of collecting urine in the clinic is recorded in the acknowledgements of publications in this period, in which scientists express their thanks to the staffs of hospitals for collecting urine: see Callow and Callow (1938). The Amsterdam School collected pregnant women's urine at the gynecological clinic of one of the city hospitals, Het Wilhelmina Gasthuis: see letter from Elisabeth Dingemanse to Ernst Laqueur, 7 February 1924, Archive Laqueur, Organon.

10 Doisy described how he collected urine with the help of a nurse in the outpatient clinic of St Louis University School of Medicine, who gave each obstetric patient a one-gallon bottle with instructions to fill it with urine and bring it on her next trip to the clinic. Later, when more urine was needed, Doisy had to deliver and collect two-gallon bottles from the homes of obstetric patients himself – a time-consuming task: see Doisy (1972: 701).

11 The German research group that had successfully isolated female sex hormones obtained large quantities of pregnancy urine from the German pharmaceutical company Schering-Kahlbaum AG: see Butenandt (1979).

12 Organon continued to supply mares' urine all through the 1950s: see Tausk (1978: 116).

13 Although biochemists became increasingly involved in the study of sex hormones, practices differed in different places. In the USA the biochemists largely worked as "handmaidens" to other scientists. Biochemists worked in other scientists' labs, often on grant money and not as salaried faculty: see Kohler (1982).

14 Source: letter from E. Laqueur to the Ministry of Defence dated 31 March 1930.

15 Source: correspondence from E. Laqueur, letters dated 14 October 1929; 7 and 12 December 1929; 31 March 1930; Archive Laqueur, Organon.

16 Many publications of these years include acknowledgements in which scientists

express their gratitude for the provision of male sex hormones. Companies often mentioned include the Schering Corporation (Germany) and Ciba Pharmaceutical Products (Switzerland): see Kochakian (1938: 463); Tschopp (1935: 1068); Warren (1935: 234). As had happened in research on female sex hormones, scientists tried once more to obtain male sex hormones from the gonads after the successful adventure with urine. In 1935 the Amsterdam School reported the isolation from tons of bull testes of 15 mg of a pure substance to which they gave the name "testosterone." Soon thereafter, this compound could be produced synthetically as well: see Tausk (1978: 89).

17 If we consider the number of publications included in the *Quarterly Cumulative Index Medicus* as an indication of progress, research on male sex hormones became substantial only after 1936, the period when scientists were no longer handicapped by a scarcity of research material. From 1927 to 1936 the number of publications on male sex hormones included in the *Quarterly Cumulative Index Medicus* varied between 2 and 35. After 1936 the number of publications increased from 28 in 1936 to 140 in 1937 and 222 in 1938.

18 The number of publications on female sex hormones indexed in the *Quarterly Cumulative Index Medicus* gradually increased from 80 in 1927 to 448 in 1938. The total number of publications in the period between 1927 and 1938 on female and male sex hormones was 2,688 and 585 respectively.

19 The medical speciality of andrology – the study of the physiology and pathology of the male reproductive system (and in this respect the counterpart of gynecology) – emerged in the 1960s. The first andrological journal (*Andrologie*) was founded in 1969. The first andrological society is either the Nordic Association for Andrology or the American Association of Andrology, both of which were established in 1973: see Niemi (1987). Clinics specializing in male reproductive functions are still very rare: andrology is usually a part of urology departments. Moreover, there still exist vast differences in the use of gynecological clinics and andrological clinics. The routine use of gynecological clinics by women, including for regular Pap smears, provides clinicians with access to large numbers of women. A routine use of andrological clinics by men has not yet developed due to the lack of any regular screening program for men (for example for prostate cancer). So in addition to the institutionalisation of specialties, the introduction of screening programs may also differentiate the access to research materials derived from the body of women and men.

20 In an interview in 1981 the German gynecologist Eberhard Nieschlag, director of the Gynecological Clinic of the Max-Planck-Gesellschaft in Münster, compared the progress in fundamental research on male reproduction with the position of research on female reproduction at the time of the First World War: see Kohaus-Altmeyer (1981).

5 THE MARKETING OF SEX HORMONES

1 The so-called Strong Program in science studies introduced the interest model, focussing the attention on the impact of professional interests, macrosociological structures, and power relations on the production and acceptance of scientific theories, results and approaches. This research program claims that scientific theories that are coincident with the economic or political interests of powerful groups are more likely to be accepted than scientific theories coincident with the interests of less powerful groups. The major representatives of the Strong Program are Barry Barnes and David Bloor: see Barnes (1977; 1985); Bloor (1976; 1983).

2 Marius Tausk, the medical director of Organon, described this strategy on the occasion of the twenty-fifth anniversary of Organon in 1948:

> From the beginning, the leading principle of Organon was not to recommend her preparations to the medical world, but only to inform the general practitioner about the nature and the application of her preparations, as objectively as possible. For, what serious doctor would be guided in the treatment of his patients by other than scientific points of view? Scientific guidelines can once only be derived from facts and observations, not from recommendations and claims.
>
> (Tausk 1948: 1)

In practice, Organon's aim to profile itself as an objective informant in the field of hormones was not unproblematic. Marius Tausk described these problems in 1935: "The problems in providing guidelines have been increased by the fact that – in our attempts to simplify the therapeutic guidelines – we could easily be suspected of simply trying to recommend specific preparations" (Tausk 1935: 1). Obviously, Organon had to justify its position as an objective informer continuously.

3 The results of these analyses were reported to general practitioners and chemists. Moreover, the institute also provided the medical profession with critical reviews of the literature on drugs, signalling "unreliable and dangerous drugs," and thus "actively participating in the fight against quackery with drugs" (Anonymous 1920). In the United States drug regulation was already institutionalized in the first decade of the twentieth century. In 1902 the US Congress passed the Biologics Control Act and in 1906 the Pure Food and Drug Act. In 1905 the American Medical Association established the Council on Pharmacy and Chemistry to set standards for drugs: see Swann (1988: 35).

4 Organon's strategy to present itself as a science-based company was not unique. In the USA

> many of the leading pharmaceutical companies were projecting a scientific image as early as the 1890s. Pharmaceutical companies began to employ medical men and maintain laboratories for quality control, standardization and product development. By the first decade of the 20th century, many American pharmaceutical firms had become science-based. Many of their products emerged from the laboratory and they conducted their advertizing campaign in scientific terms.
>
> (Liebenau 1987: 4, 79)

5 Recommended by Laqueur as a scientific name, *Menformon* was adopted by Organon as a trade name – a rather unusual practice, because scientific names were normally restricted to scientific use: see Tausk (1978: 31–32).

6 Source: interview with Dr Ina Uyldert, 2 December 1987.

7 According to Tausk, pharmaceutical companies could market their products without any preceding clinical trials. The Inspection of Public Health and the Food and Drug Administration did not (yet) control the products of drug manufacturers: see Tausk (1978: 32).

8 The patents of this early period proved to be of no practical value in the years to follow. Organon dropped these patents in 1934: see Tausk (1978: 111).

9 In the late 1930s Organon also requested the cooperation of physicians. In 1937 Organon described the need to cooperate with physicians:

> The pharmaceutical industry and the pharmacologist are not equipped to determine the usefulness of hormone preparations. Only the physicians can contribute to obtaining a better judgement about the therapeutic significance

of the preparations which are delivered to them, by systematically and critically collecting or reporting the results obtained.

(Tausk 1937: 6)

10 In Laqueur's correspondence there are regular accounts of contacts with gynecological clinics in order to arrange for the collection of raw materials as well as the organization of clinical trials (Organon Archive 26 March, 2 May and 14 July 1927; 4 October 1928).

11 In the early 1930s the dosage of female sex hormone therapy was a topic of debate. In 1932 Marius Tausk described the practice of female sex hormone therapy, criticizing the enormous variability in quantities, varying from 4 to 4,000 units of female sex hormone. Tausk interpreted these variations in doses as resulting from failures in treatment leading to an increase of the dosage, and from the different purposes of the therapy: see Tausk (1932b: 15). In the late 1930s the dosage of female sex hormones became once again a topic of debate. This time the discussion was fueled by the suggestion that the use of large doses could cause cancer.

12 The injection of female sex hormones required a lower dosage than oral administration. This difference in dosage provided Organon with the major advantage that the same quantity of raw material could be used for the production of much larger quantities of female sex hormone preparations (in the form of injections) than its previous products (tablets) (Dongen 1929). During the 1920s and 1930s the clinical results of female sex hormone therapy remained unstable, partly as a result of the differences in the raw materials from which sex hormones were prepared. In the early decades commercial preparations consisted primarily of powder from whole ovaries. In the 1920s most products consisted of extracts of the ovaries, while in the 1930s urine had become the major raw material for the production of female sex hormones. These products not only varied in terms of the quantity of active substance, but also differed in the quality of the ingredient, possibly even containing different chemical substances.

13 After the detection of female sex hormone in the urine of pregnant women in 1927, the manufacturing of *Menformon* became less expensive and the production of hormone preparations was far less constrained by the limited availability of raw materials. Consequently, *Menformon* became available in larger quantities than the previous product. The cooperation with the clinics provided Organon with the required amounts of female urine. As we saw in Chapter 4, the constraints on the production of female sex hormone due to the limited availability of raw materials was finally solved in 1930. The availability of mares' urine as a new source, and the introduction of a quantitative test to determine the content of female sex hormones in the urine (by the Dutch chemist Kober), enabled Organon to increase their production of female sex hormone preparations enormously: see Tausk (1978: 35, 116, 117).

14 Organon Archive, January 1925 (undated letter).

15 Laqueur chose the methodology of double-blind trials in a historical period in which the use of experimental controls was not yet standard practice in clinical experimentation. The use of "objectively measured indicators of response to treatment and blinded assessments of therapeutic outcomes" became adopted in clinical experimentation only in the latter half of the twentieth century: see Marks (1987a: 35; 1987b: 154).

16 Laqueur described this construction of hormone deficiency as a specific illness:

Organ and hormone preparations are mostly applied in cases of a deficiency of one or the other substance: as substitute-therapy. The indication for sex hormones, however, is quite unfavorable. The seriousness of the diseases caused by deficiency of these hormones is usually not such that danger to life is involved and one could save patients by administration of sex hormones, as in the case of insulin. . . . A deficiency of sex hormones, however, causes very unpleasant symptoms, and the number of people suffering from this without being actually sick in the usual sense of the word, is much larger than those who are said to be really ill.

(Laqueur 1937)

17 As in the case of menopausal disorders, economic incentives also played a role in research on menstruation. In the 1920s scientists investigated the economic meaning of menstruation. In Britain the Industrial Fatigue Research Board investigated whether "the female body, being subject to periodic change, has any harmful drawbacks for her activities in industry or professions" (Pinkhof 1928: 1,948).

18 In the 1980s estrogen replacement therapy provided the major market for estrogen administration, in particular in the United States: see Kaufert and McKinlay (1987: 113–139).

19 *Acta Brevia Neerlandica* was founded by Ernst Laqueur in order to provide a journal for short communications on the development of endocrinological research. In this journal Laqueur could publish his research results within a rather short period. This was particularly relevant to guarantee specific research results to his credit in order to claim the right of patent. Source: interview with Dr. Ina Uyldert, 2 December 1987.

20 In 1934 de Jongh had already published the results of experiments with rats in which the incubation of the ova was prevented by injections with *Menformon*: see Jongh (1934a: 731).

21 In The Netherlands Aletta Jacobs and Johannes Rutgers were the first physicians who strongly advocated and practiced medical assistance in birth control. As early as 1878, Rutgers had founded the world's first birth control clinic in Amsterdam. This clinic was run by volunteers because Rutgers did not receive any cooperation from his medical colleagues: see Emde Boas (1933: 416).

22 At the beginning of the twentieth century, Dutch politicians, churches and the feminist movement all strongly opposed birth control. In 1911 the Dutch government (under a confessional cabinet, that is exclusively Catholics and Protestants) passed a law against the exhibition, advertisement or propaganda of contraception. Only after 1920 did opinions shift, although the real breakthrough did not happen until after the Second World War. In the late 1930s many Dutch general practitioners had gradually adopted the arguments of the Dutch Neo-Malthusians, who had advocated birth control since the turn of the century: see Outshoorn (1979: 60–73). Obviously, the changing attitude toward contraception was rather fragile, since Organon and Dutch gynecologists were very restrictive in developing research on hormonal contraceptives. Even after the Second World War, Dutch gynecologists kept their restrictive attitude toward contraception. Danning and de Snoo, two leading Dutch gynecologists, then campaigned against the import of contraceptives in The Netherlands: see Schoon (1990: 78).

23 This test consisted of a bio-assay in which the urine of women was injected into young female mice. If this injection caused hemorrhaging in the ovaries, the test indicated the presence of a gonadotropic hormone, originating from the placenta, and excreted in large amounts during pregnancy: see Tausk (1931: 14).

24 For a description of the testicular transplantation practice in the early decades of the twentieth century, see Hamilton (1986: 18–19).

25 The male menopause also included symptoms other than sexual impotence.

In 1938, Marius Tausk described the male climacterium as "a decline in potency, accompanied by symptoms like blood pressure in the head, sleeplessness, psychological depression, feelings of anxiety and a decline in work power." In this article Tausk is rather skeptical about the effectiveness of male sex hormone treatment, emphasizing the importance of psychological causes and the possibility of suggestive rather than rational effects of male sex hormone therapy (Tausk 1938b: 131–136).

26 The subject of clinical trials with male sex hormones in psychiatric clinics is addressed only twice in the correspondence of Laqueur.

27 Clinical trials with these combined preparations are mentioned in the letters in Organon's Archive dated 20 April and 17 November 1932; 2 October 1936.

28 Tausk did not give any reason why testosterone therapy was not suitable as a replacement for female sex hormone therapy. Following the conceptualization of male sex hormones as agents controlling masculinity, the expectation that the prescription of male sex hormones might lead to the "masculinization" of female patients may have been a possible motive. Although other authors suggested these possible "side-effects," particularly in the case of high dosages of male sex hormone, Tausk did not refer to these effects (Tausk 1938b: 132, 133, 135; 1939a).

29 The debate on cancer and DES was reopened again in the 1970s, when American scientists published reports on the incidence of cancer in children of "DES mothers," women treated with DES during pregnancy to prevent miscarriages: see Groenewegen *et al.* (1988).

30 For a more recent case-study of drugs development, in which drugs are depicted in this way, see Vos 1989.

31 Personal communication of Adele Clarke.

6 THE TRANSFORMATION OF SEX HORMONES INTO THE PILL

1 "All the conventional contraceptives depended upon setting up a mechanical or chemical barrier to prevent sperm cells from reaching the egg cells" (Maisel 1965: 114).

2 See among others Knorr-Cetina (1981a; 1981b); Pinch (1985).

3 In 1873 the US Congress had enacted legislation that prohibited mailing, transporting or importing "obscene, lewd, and lascivious" articles. All contraceptive devices were included in these statutes, known as the Comstock Laws, which were designed to preserve the purity of late Victorian life in the United States. Moreover, many state laws stated that no one could give out information on contraception to anyone for any reason. Although the majority of the Comstock Laws were repealed in the post-Second World War period of retreat from prudery, many state laws prohibiting the dissemination of contraceptive information functioned well into the 1960s; for an extensive description of these laws see Ward (1986: 6). Moreover, the statutes were not restricted to forbidding the dissemination of contraceptive information, but went even further, making a crime of the "use of drugs or instruments to prevent conception" (Rock 1963: 107).

4 For a thorough analysis of the controversial status of reproductive research, see Clarke (1990b). Clarke distinguished four domains of controversy that shaped the development of the reproductive sciences in the USA: "association with sexuality and reproduction; association with quackery; association with controversial social movements; and the capacity of the reproductive sciences to create Brave New Worlds" (Clarke 1990b: 26).

5 Physicians also gradually opposed the restrictive attitude toward birth control.

In 1937, after two decades of campaigning by the feminist Margaret Sanger, the American Medical Association agreed to support birth control: see Ward (1986: 8). In the 1930s and 1940s there were several attempts by physicians to change the Comstock Laws that banned the dissemination of all information about fertility limitations, medical information included. They tried, in vain, to get this restriction on medical practice removed from the law: see Rock (1963: 75).

6 One of the ironies of the birth control movement is the ideological shift from the view that women should be given control over their fertility as a step to a better quality of life to the conservative stand that birth control should be used for eugenic and population control concerns: see Ward (1986: 8). For an extensive study of how the feminist ideology of individual rights and sexual freedom gradually disappeared from the agenda of the birth control movement, see Borell (1987); Gordon (1976).

7 Sanger believed that the most important threat to women's independence came from unwanted and unanticipated pregnancies. She advocated birth control as a basic precondition to the liberation of women: see Christian Johnson (1977: 1). Sanger was the founder of the American Birth Control League in 1920, which joined the Planned Parenthood Federation in the 1940s; she was arrested and jailed for opening the first birth control clinic in New York in 1916: see Maisel (1965: 207).

8 Pincus initiated and chaired the major yearly conference on hormones (the Laurentian Hormone Conference) and was editor of *Progress in Hormone Research* for many years: see Maisel (1965: 111).

9 Pincus was already familiar with the pharmaceutical world. After his departure from Harvard, he had worked as a special consultant on a contractual basis for many pharmaceutical companies in the USA and Mexico: see McLaughlin (1982: 112).

10 As expressed by Oscar Hechter, a biologist and one of Pincus's colleagues at the Worcester Foundation: see Anonymous (1978: 16).

11 In later years Pincus became one of the major advocates of hormonal contraceptives, traveling all over the world to propagate these contraceptives as a means to solve the "population problem." In *The Control of Fertility* he described how he "had faced the hard fact of overpopulation in country after country, learned of the bleak demographic future, assessed the prospects for the practice of efficient fertility control" (Pincus 1965: viii).

12 McCormick as cites in Seaman and Seaman (1977: 145).

13 In the 1930s and 1940s Pincus and Rock had worked together in a research project on test-tube fertilization. They had lost touch in the 1940s: see McLaughlin (1982: 41, 108).

14 Rock's studies were based on the theory that infertility might be related to an underdevelopment of the tubes and womb. The administration of progesterone (and estrogens) was expected to stimulate the growth of these organs and thus facilitate fertilization and pregnancy (Rock 1963: 163).

15 Actually, this decision meant a crucial turn for both Rock's career and his personal life. Rock considered himself a scrupulous Catholic and was fully aware of the fact that he would cooperate in a research project that was diametrically opposed to the Church's dogma that opposed all "unnatural" means of contraception. In *The Pill, John Rock and the Church* McLaughlin (1982) described how Rock's Catholic background interacted with his scientific work. During his whole career Rock tried to reconcile these conflicting domains. Rock's reputation as a Catholic and a leading gynecologist made him an ideal person to bridge these two worlds. This played an important role in the eventual acceptance of contraceptives. Rock gradually became a major

advocate for the production of better birth control methods and, in the 1960s, the pill. In 1963, he published *The Time Has Come: A Catholic Doctor's Proposals to End the Battle over Birth Control*. In this book Rock chose a position as Catholic and as scientist in the ongoing dispute over birth control, and called for a "Manhattan Project" for contraceptive research: see Piotrow (1973: 76); Rock (1963).

16 At the time of Pincus's request, Searle's laboratories were already involved in a search for an orally active progestin, which resulted eventually in the synthesis of what were called 19 nor-steroids. The initial work on orally effective progestins was done in order to develop a drug for the treatment of cervical cancer (Anonymous 1978: 33). Actually, Syntex was the first to manufacture 19 nor-steroids and patented the first oral progestin as early as 1951 as a drug for the treatment of menstrual problems: see Seaman and Seaman (1977: 65).

17 This practice of testing raises questions about whether the women were informed about the purpose of the tests. They were not. This experiment, and later experiments in which side-effects of the progestins were investigated, "violated two basic tenets of informed consent in medical research – that subjects be given a full explanation of the nature, duration, and purpose of the study and a description of discomfort and risks" (Ramirez de Arellano and Seipp 1983: 117). In this period, however, there was very little development of any formal informed consent, that is "a patient's right to be knowledgeable about a proposed treatment and to have a meaningful choice whether to submit to that treatment" (Barber 1980: 35). Serious informed consent procedures were not developed until the 1960s. In Europe, the concept of informed consent was first discussed in 1945 following the discovery that

> Nazi doctors had experimented without their consent on prisoners in the concentration camps. As a result of the trial and imprisonment of these doctors, the Nuremburg Code for experimentation on any subjects, which was formulated in 1947, explicitly stated the requirement of informed consent.
>
> (Barber 1980: 29–30)

In the USA informed consent protocols were introduced in 1962 triggered by malpractice cases (particularly abuse of research on black men, retarded and insane people, and prisoners) and the thalidomide tragedy (Barber 1980: 42, 155). The concept of informed consent was formally adopted by the medical profession in 1964 in the Declaration of Helsinki. "Many world, national, and professional specialty codes for experimentation have been published since then, and all emphasize the importance of informed consent" (Barber 1980: 30, 341). Despite these regulations, there still exists the abuse of women in clinical trials of contraceptives such as the more recently developed long-acting hormone injectables and subdermal implants.

> Reports from several countries such as Bangladesh, India, Peru, and Thailand all show that the women involved in trials are rarely told that the hormonal contraceptives being given to them are in the trial phase, or, that they may cause serious short- and long-term adverse effects in health.
>
> (Gupta 1991: 93)

18 The bleedings, however, were quite different from bleedings without the pill. In their publications, the authors kept referring to these bleedings as menstrual flow: see e.g. Pincus (1959: 309).

19 The fact that scientists emphasize the naturalness of their products is not specific to the pill. Presenting drugs as natural is a strategy that is often used

in the introduction of new drugs. In the case of the pill, the argument of naturalness was used not only as a strategy toward consumers, but also to convince the Catholic opponents of the pill that this new type of contraceptive was not in conflict with the Church ideology that opposed all "unnatural" means of contraception.

20 The occurrence of negative side-effects was a controversial issue that was debated until far into the 1970s: see also note 37.

21 Rock considered the results of the trials too premature for a presentation at a conference. Moreover, he was well aware of the negative opinions of many leading clinicians toward contraception and, only a year away from retirement, he did not want to jeopardize a long and distinguished career. Another reason was that Rock did not want to harden the opposition of the Church. After he retired from Harvard, Rock moved his practice into new quarters and founded the Rock Reproductive Center, somewhat more independent from the opinion and judgement of the Harvard medical establishment. In 1955, McCormick financed the renovation of this new clinic: see McLaughlin (1982: 116, 121).

22 Laws prohibiting birth control were repealed as early as 1937 due to successful lobbying of the birth control movement in Puerto Rico (Ramirez de Arellano and Seipp 1983: 21, 29, 49, 94); see also note 29.

23 David Tyler to Gregory Pincus, 8 July 1955 (cited in Ramirez de Arellano and Seipp 1983: 110).

24 The Worcester Foundation for Experimental Biology "had long-standing ties to the mental hospital through Mrs. McCormick, who had established the Neuroendocrine Research Foundation there in 1927. McCormick paid the hospital to modernize the experimental wards" (McLaughlin 1982: 119).

25 While not noted in the historical materials, the hospital director may have been willing to participate because pregnancy due to sexual assault and abuse has been common in hospitals for insane and mentally handicapped people. Personal communication from Adele Clarke.

26 Feminists have suggested that side-effects of contraceptives in men have been treated far more seriously than the side-effects of contraceptives in women: see Seaman and Seaman (1977: 70–71).

27 The "conspiracy of silence," to use Sanger's words, was definitely broken in 1958 when Pincus and Rock published the results of the first field trials. In the *American Journal of Obstetrics and Gynecology*, they first deliberately used a title that explicitly expressed the topic of their research: "Fertility Control with Oral Medication." The 1959 publication in *Science* entitled "Effectiveness of an Oral Contraceptive," definitely lifted the veil from their contraceptive research project.

28 The problem of finding suitable, motivated research subjects was not specific for the testing of the pill. Clinical investigators in other areas are sometimes confronted with similar problems. For another example see Fox (1959). There were, however, certain aspects in which the testing of the pill was rather peculiar. In contrast with the testing of other drugs, this testing required assessment of healthy women. Consequently, investigators could not rely on hospitalized patients but needed to create an infrastructure in which the testing could take place.

29 The Puerto Rican birth control and family planning movement has a long history that can be traced back to the 1920s. The first birth control organization, the Birth Control League, was founded as early as 1925, but disbanded again in 1928 due to the same restrictive laws that constrained the birth control movement in the continental United States. The Birth Control League had close connections with the birth control movements in the USA and The Netherlands. The league sought the help of Margaret Sanger and relied on

the writings of Dr Aletta Jacobs, a Dutch physician who had opened a contraceptive clinic in Amsterdam as early as 1882. In 1932, the Birth Control League opened its first clinic in San Juan and began providing contraceptive services. In 1936, the birth control movement first created strong ties to the medical profession and constituted the Maternal and Child Health Association, with professors of the University of Puerto Rico as members. The association opened three clinics. All these efforts lasted only a short time due to the lack of political support. This situation changed in 1937 as a result of successful lobbying of the birth control movement for the repeal of the Puerto Rican Comstock Laws. Legislation enabling the dissemination of contraceptive information and practices was approved in April of that year. After this liberalization of the Puerto Rican law, the organization of large-scale birth control programs no longer met with legal opposition. The birth control movement became institutionalized as a formal, politically accepted organization in 1946 with the foundation of the Population Association, consisting of university professors as well as government officials. In 1953, the Population Association was renamed the Family Planning Association: see Ramirez de Arellano and Seipp (1983: 21, 29, 49, 94).

30 At the end of the Spanish–American War in 1898, Puerto Rico changed its status from a Spanish colony into a US colony. The island was of military significance for the USA because of its geographic location and was considered as "the Gibraltar of the Caribbean." Even today large parts of the island are still the property of the United States' armed forces and are used, among other things, for missile tracking stations as well as a training ground for the Peace Corps. Puerto Rico remained under the jurisdiction of the US War Department until 1934. In 1952, the island received the status of a "commonwealth," a "free associated state" of the USA. This meant a far greater measure of political autonomy than it had previously enjoyed, including

> the right to draft its own constitutions, to select its governor by popular election, and exercise authority in all spheres except the military, the federal judiciary, and foreign affairs. Puerto Ricans continued to be citizens of the U.S. but had no voting representation in the Congress neither the right to participate in national elections.
>
> (Ramirez de Arellano and Seipp 1983: 4, 6, 89–90)

31 Indeed, the testing of the pill was not the first time that Puerto Rico was used as a location for contraceptive research. In 1936, the US Birth Control League had chosen Puerto Rico with its birth control clinics as the ideal site to test contraceptive methods such as diaphragms and contraceptive jellies. One year later, the chemical firm Johnson and Johnson cooperated with the Maternal and Child Health Association to test a spermicidal powder: see Ramirez de Arellano and Seipp (1983: 45, 47). Moreover, Puerto Rico has been the site of an extensive experimentation and use of sterilization, starting in the late 1930s. In 1935, the Puerto Rican Medical Association "persuaded its colleagues to approve a resolution requesting legislative action to permit the teaching and demonstration of contraceptive methods and the sterilization of the mentally deficient" (Ramirez de Arellano and Seipp (1983: 41–42). The first surgical sterilizations were performed at the "highly reputable" Presbyterian Hospital in San Juan, which added to the respectability and prestige of this contraceptive method. The medical profession in Puerto Rico welcomed sterilization "as an opportunity for the practice of surgical skills." Despite severe religious and political protests, "*la operacion*" developed into a widespread contraceptive practice and was advocated by "mainland eugenists" as the solution to Puerto Rico's "reckless overbreeding." In the late 1940s, sterilizations of women who

had already given birth to a number of children were being carried out "almost as a routine procedure" and sterilization had become "a somewhat common mode of birth control in Puerto Rico" (Ramirez de Arellano and Seipp 1983: 135–138). Sadly enough, the history of sterilization shows that there has been much abuse of women, in Puerto Rico and elsewhere, in which women were even sterilized without their knowledge: see Gupta (1991: 105).

32 Sanger to McCormick, 27 October 1950 (cited in Christian Johnson 1977: 67). Since the early 1920s Sanger had visited many Third World countries to explain the contribution that birth control could make toward reducing poverty: see Gordon (1976: 336).

33 Since the early 1940s Puerto Rico had witnessed a high increase of its population due to a remarkable improvement in the health of its residents, leading to a decrease in death rate to a percentage that was even lower than that of the continental USA (Ramirez de Arellano and Seipp 1983: 84).

34 For an extensive study of how birth control became intertwined with governmental policies and gradually developed into population control as a form of cultural imperialism, see Gordon (1976). Many liberal governments of underdeveloped countries, including Puerto Rican nationalists, perceived the birth control programs as a means of deflecting attention from the real problems. They ascribed the causes of underdevelopment to colonialism and cultural imperialism. In their view, overpopulation might have contributed to poverty, but it was definitely not the cause. Poverty should be cured by economic development (Gordon 1976: 336–337). The two opposing views, "development as the best contraceptive" versus "contraception as the best developmental tool," are still uttered in debates about birth control in Third World countries (Ramirez de Arellano and Seipp 1983: 180).

35 Pincus was not alone in considering Puerto Rico a promising location for research. Since the 1940s, its people have been the subjects of numerous research projects. Puerto Rico, easily accessible as a former colony of the United States, functioned as a laboratory for demographers and other social scientists. It became the USA's "showcase of development" (Ramirez de Arellano and Seipp 1983: 62, 94, 88, 174). "Probably nowhere in the world has a society been as extensively observed, enumerated, and assessed as in Puerto Rico" (Ramirez de Arellano and Seipp 1983: ix).

36 The trial in Port-au-Prince in Haiti was started at the invitation of "Papa Doc" Duvalier, who was persuaded that a birth control program would be profitable for the economics of the island. The political situation in Haiti led to the failure of this trial.

> The Boston team became alarmed when they discovered that the medical system was under political control and were shocked by the tendency of people involved in the trial to disappear suddenly, including the chief administrator, a former chief of the Haitian Air Force. In 1969 only one member of the original committee of four survived and the records of the project were in a state of irreversible confusion.
>
> (Vaughan 1972: 55)

37 Side-effects of the pill also remained a controversial issue after the Puerto Rican trials had ended. The most heated controversy emerged in the early 1960s when reports were published that the pill caused thromboembolism: a blood clot in the vein. In the late 1960s, feminists and health advocates campaigned against the side-effects of the pill and accused the medical profession and the pharmaceutical industry of not seriously considering the many complaints of pill users (Seaman 1969). In 1969, the *Lancet* concluded in an editorial that

the metabolic changes associated with this treatment may modify biochemical processes in all body tissues. More than 50 metabolic changes have been recorded. . . . These changes are unnecessary for contraception and the ultimate effect on the health of the user is unknown . . . the wisdom of administering such compounds to healthy women for many years must be questioned seriously.

(as cited in Seaman and Seaman 1977: x)

Not until 1981 did pharmaceutical firms introduce a hormonal oral contraceptive that did not have the side-effects of the previous pills (Breedeveld 1992).

38 Pincus as cited in Seaman (1969: 182).
39 McCormick as cited in McLaughlin (1982: 132).
40 The role of the FDA at that time was different from today. In the 1960s the FDA did not yet have the power to refuse admittance of new drugs because of safety concerns. Then the FDA's work focussed on quality control in the purity of manufacturing any new drugs. If safety was taken into account, the burden of proof was on the side of the FDA and not on the side of the drug companies: see McLaughlin (1982: 141); Seaman (1969: 182). Drug legislation in the USA changed considerably in response to the thalidomide tragedy. In 1961, the drug thalidomide was identified as the source of the outbreak of phocomelia, a condition where children are born without hands or feet. In the USA, thalidomide had been distributed to doctors in the context of clinical testing. The FDA, however, "did not have the authority to supervise the clinical testing of drugs. The 1962 Drug Amendments gave the FDA increasing control over the approval of drugs. The testing of drugs like thalidomide could thereby no longer be undertaken without prior notification of the FDA."

Besides changing the standards for approving a new drug, it made the FDA into an active participant in the approval process. Instead of letting a firm's New Drug Approval (NDA) take effect automatically if the FDA did not object, the new law required affirmative FDA approval before marketing could begin. In addition, the amendments gave the FDA jurisdiction over the testing of all new drugs before they were approved for marketing. A drug firm had to apply to the FDA for approval of its procedures for testing an investigational new drug before it could undertake the tests needed to file an NDA.

(Temin 1980: 123, 125)

Some authors have suggested that the FDA would never have granted its approval for the testing and the marketing of the first oral contraceptive if the pill had been introduced after the thalidomide disaster took place (Anonymous 1978: 15).

41 I. C. Winter, Searle's executive (cited in McLaughlin 1982: 139).
42 This trial, carried out by Edward Tyler, a gynecologist who was acquainted with Pincus, was not constrained by any laws because the Comstock Laws were already repealed in this state: see Vaughan (1972: 55–56). Although the ethnic background of the participants is not described in the trial reports, it is very likely, given the multiracial population of Los Angeles, that black and Hispanic women participated in this trial.
43 Throughout the 1960s, Puerto Rico continued to serve as a laboratory for the testing of new contraceptives, including new brands and generations of hormonal oral contraceptives, hormonal skin-deposits, vaginal foams and intrauterine devices: see Ramirez de Arellano and Seipp (1983: 131).
44 I would like to thank Diana Long, who clarified this point to me.

45 See among others hooks (1982).

7 THE POWER OF STRUCTURES THAT ALREADY EXIST

1 I draw here specifically on the conceptual work of social constructivist studies of science and technology: see for instance Latour (1987); Pinch and Bijker (1987). The terms recontextualization and decontextualization are used, among others, by Knorr-Cetina (1981a; 1981b).

2 The theme of local versus universal knowledge has been addressed, among others, by Star (1989).

3 The concept of the configured user has been introduced by Woolgar (1992).

4 Such regular medical examinations of pill users were normal medical practice in all countries in which the pill was introduced until the mid-1980s.

5 Contraceptive injectables (like *Depo Provera*) have an efficacy period of at least three months, and consequently have to be repeated at least every three months; most of its users live in developing countries: see Hardon (1992: 12). Contraceptive implants (like *Norplant*) are long-acting methods (five years) which must be inserted under the skin of a woman's upper arm and removed by a health care worker. The introduction of this contraceptive method in developing countries is highly controversial: see Mintzes (1992).

6 This emphasis on user-controlled contraceptive technologies is not unproblematic. From this perspective, feminist health activists tend to reject injectable or subdermal techniques, although these same techniques are favored by women in Indonesia, for example. This preference is apparently related to the fact that these methods can more easily be kept hidden from partners, who do not agree with their decision to practice birth control: see Hardon and Claudio-Estrada (1991: 12).

7 Introductory trials were first used in the assessment of the acceptability of *Norplant*. These trials, however, seem to have similar flaws. Health advocates suggest that introductory trials are rather limited in scope and perspective.

> They are done in controlled settings and include women who have been carefully selected and thus are not representative of the whole population that eventually will use a method. They generally do not study all effects, including social and economical effects, which are important to the users of contraceptives.
>
> (Hardon 1992: 18)

8 This shift from the gonads to the brain was further reinforced in the late 1950s, when neuro-endocrinologists introduced the so-called 'organizational theory,' a theory that explains sexual differentiation in terms of the relation between prenatal hormones and brain development. For an extensive analysis of this field, see Wijngaard (1991b).

9 In this paper, Anne Fausto-Sterling described the medical treatment of intersexuality. Since the 1960s, intersexual children, that is children who are born with both male and female reproductive organs (approximately 4 per cent of all births) receive surgical and hormonal treatment in such a way that these children are 'generally squeezed into one of the two prevailing categories,' thus erasing 'any embodied sex that does not conform to a male-female, heterosexual pattern.' For another critical analysis of the medical treatment of intersexual children, see Wijngaard (1991b).

10 The association of femininity with cyclicity became widespread particularly after the 1960s, when gynecologists and physicians reintroduced the Premenstrual Syndrome. In this diagnostic category, female reproductive functions

became linked with behavioral categories, in a process whereby femininity became increasingly associated with instability and unreliability: see Branssen (1988: 28–43).

11 I thank Adele Clarke, who introduced this term to me.

Bibliography

Aberle, S.D., Corner, G.W. (1953) *Twenty-five Years of Sex Research: History of the National Research Council Committee for Research in Problems of Sex 1922–1947*, Philadelphia, Pa and London: W.B. Saunders.

Akrich, M. (1992) "The De-scription of Technological Objects," in Bijker, W.E., Law, J. (eds) *Shaping Technology – Building Society*, Cambridge, Mass.: MIT Press.

Alcoff, L. (1988) "Cultural Feminism versus Poststructuralism: The Identity Crisis in Feminist Theory," *Signs: Journal of Women in Culture and Society* 13 (3): 405–436.

Allen, E., Hisaw, F.L., Gardner, W.U. (1939) "The Endocrine Function of the Ovaries," in E. Allen (ed.) *Sex and Internal Secretions*, 2nd edn, Baltimore, Md: William & Wilkins.

Amsterdamska, O. (1987) "Medical and Biological Constraints: Early Research on Variation in Bacteriology," *Social Studies of Science* 17: 657–687.

Anonymous (1920) "Pharmaco-Therapeutisch Instituut", *Nederlands Tijdschrift voor Geneeskunde* 64: 1,435–1,475

—— (1937) *Zaklexicon der Orgaan- en Hormoontherapie*, Tweede herziene uitgave, Organon.

—— (1938) *Wie is dat?*, 's-Gravenhage: Martinus Nijhoff.

—— (1978) "Historical Perspectives on the Scientific Study of Fertility," Transcript from the Conference on Historical Perspectives of the Scientific Study of Fertility, Session III. The Development of Endocrinology, American Academy of Arts and Sciences, Boston, Mass., 5 May 1978.

—— (1985) *The Depo-Provera Debate: A Report by the National Women's Health Network*, Washington, DC: National Women's Health Network.

—— (1992) "Vrouwen stappen over op oude, goedkope pil," *Nieuwe Rotterdamse Courant*, 16 January.

Atkinson, L.E., Lincoln, R., Forest., J.D. (1985) "Worldwide Trends in Funding for Contraceptive Research and Evaluation," *Family Planning Perspectives* 17: 196–207.

Baart, I., Bransen, E. (1986) "Waar eens de baarmoeder raasde. Wetenschappelijke waarheid en medische theorievorming," *Lover* 13: (1): 4–14.

Back, R.H., Stycos, J.M. (1962) "Population Control in Puerto Rico: The Formal and the Informal Framework," *Law and Contemporary Problems* 11: 558–576.

Banta, D.H., Behney, C.J. (1981) "Policy Formulation and Technology Assessment," *Milbank Memorial Fund Quarterly: Health and Society* 59: 445–479.

Barber, B. (1980) *Informed Consent in Medical Therapy and Research*, New Brunswick, NJ: Rutgers University Press.

Barnes, B. (1977) *Interests and the Growth of Knowledge*, London: Routledge & Kegan Paul.
—— (1985) *The Nature of Power*, Oxford: Polity.
Beach, F.A. (1981) "Historical Origins of Modern Research on Hormones and Behavior," *Hormones and Behavior* 15: 325–376.
Beauchamp, T.L., Childress, J.F. (1983) *Principles of Biomedical Ethics*, 2nd edn, New York, Oxford: Oxford University Press.
Beck, E., Schmitz, G. (1936) "Therapy of Schizophrenia in Males with Progynon (female sex hormone)," *Deutsches Medisches Wochenschrift* 62: 544–545.
Beek, M. van der (1933) "Behandeling van de depressieve psychoses bij vrouwen met ovariumhormonen," *Nederlands Tijdschrift voor Geneeskunde* 77: 3,249–3,259.
Bell, B. (1916) *The Sex Complex: A Study of the Relationship of the Internal Secretions to the Female Characteristics and Functions in Health and Disease*. London: Baillière, Tindall & Cox.
Bell, S.E. (1986) "A New Model of Medical Technology Development: A Case Study of DES," *Research in the Sociology of Health Care* 4: 1–33.
—— (1987) "Changing Ideas: The Medicalization of Menopause," *Social Science and Medicine* 24: 535–542.
Belt, H. v.d., Gremmen, B. (1988) "Het specificiteitsbegrip in de tijd van Koch en Ehrlich: Een nieuwe interpretatie van de 'serologische denkstijl van Ludwik Fleck,' *Kennis en Methode* XII: 35–334.
Berg, M. (1992) "The Construction of Medical Disposals: Medical Sociology and Medical Problem Solving in Clinical Practice,' *Sociology of Health and Illness* 14: 151–180.
Bijker, W. E. (1993) "Do Not Despair: There is Life after Constructivism," *Science, Technology and Human Values* 18 (1): 113–29.
Bijker, W. E., Hughes, T. P., Pinch, T. J. (eds) (1987) *The Social Construction of Technological Systems: New Directions in the Sociology and History of Technology*, Cambridge, Mass.: MIT Press.
Bijker, W. E., Law, J. (1992) *Shaping Technology – Building Society*, Cambridge, Mass.: MIT Press.
Binsberg, C. (1949) *Female Sex Endocrinology*, Philadelphia, Pa: Lippincott.
Birke, L. (1986) *Women, Feminism and Biology: The Feminist Challenge*, Brighton, Sussex: Harvester.
Blauwhof, G., Rossum, W. van, Zeldenrust, S. (1990) "The Development of Technologies: Towards a Network Analysis"?, Key-paper prepared for the Dutch workshop on technology research, Groningen 31 May–1 June (unpublished manuscript).
Bleier, R. (1979) "Social and Political Bias in Science: An Examination of Animal Studies and their Generalizations to Human Behavior and Evolution," in E. Tobach, B. Rosoff (eds) *Genes and Gender*, New York: Pergamon.
—— (1984) *Science and Gender: A Critique of Biology and its Theories on Women*, New York: Pergamon.
—— (ed.) (1986) *Feminist Approaches to Science*, New York: Pergamon.
Bloor, D. (1976) *Knowledge and Social Imagery*, London: Routledge & Kegan Paul.
—— (1983) *A Social Theory of Knowledge*, London: Macmillan
Blume S. (1992) *Insight and Industry*, Cambridge, Mass.: MIT Press.
Bodewitz, H.J.H.W., Buurma, H., Vries, G.H. de (1987) "Regulatory Science and the Social Management of Trust in Medicine," in W.E. Bijker, T.P. Hughes, T.J. Pinch (eds) *The Social Construction of Technological Systems: New Directions in the Sociology and History of Technology*, Cambridge, Mass.: MIT Press.
Borchardt, E., Dingemanse, E., Jongh, S.E. de., Laqueur, E. (1928) "Over het

vrouwelijk geslachtshormoon Menformon, in het bijzonder over de anti-masculine werking," *Nederlands Tijdschrift Geneeskunde.* 72: 1,028.

Borell, M. (1976a) "Brown-Séquard's Organotherapy and its Appearance in America at the End of the Nineteenth Century," *Bulletin of the History of Medicine* 50: 309–320.

—— (1976b) "Organotherapy, British Physiology, and the Discovery of the Internal Secretions," *Journal of the History of Biology* 9: 235–268.

—— (1985) "Organotherapy and the Emergence of Reproductive Endocrinology," *Journal of the History of Biology* 18: 1–30.

—— (1987) "Biologists and Birth Control 1918–1938," *Journal of the History of Biology* 20: 51–87.

Braidotti, R. (1989) "Organs without Bodies," *Differences* 1: 147–162.

—— (1991) "On Contemporary Medical Pornography," *Tijdschrift voor Vrouwenstudies* 12 (3): 356–372.

Branssen, E. (1988) "Wankele wezens: Het premenstrueel syndroom en de constructie van vrouwelijkheid," *Tijdschrift voor Vrouwenstudies* 9(1): 28–43.

Breedeveld, M. (1992) "Pilfabrikant op zoek naar nieuwe markten," *Nieuwe Rotterdamse Courant* 20 October.

Brennan, T. (1992) *The Interpretation of the Flesh: Freud and Femininity,* London and New York: Routledge.

Briscoe, A.M. (1978) "Hormones and Gender," in E. Tobach, B. Rosoff (eds) *Genes and Gender,* New York: Gordian.

Bromwich, P., Parsons, T. (1990) *Contraception: The Facts,* Oxford: Oxford University Press.

Bruce, J. (1987) "Users' Perspectives on Contraceptive Technology and Delivery Systems," *Technology in Society* 9: 359–383.

Burt, R.S. (1982) *Toward a Structural Theory of Action,* New York: Academic Press.

Burt, R.S., Minor, M.J. (1983) *Applied Network Analysis,* Beverly Hills, Calif.: Sage.

Butenandt, A. (1979) "50 Years Ago: The Discovery of Oestrone," *Trends in Biochemical Sciences* 4: 215–217.

Cadbury, G.W. (1962) "Outlook for Government Action in Family Planning in the West Indies," in C.V. Kiser (ed.) *Family Planning,* Princeton, NJ: Princeton University Press.

Caldwell, W.E., Moloy, H.C., D'Esopo, D.A. (1934) "Further Studies on the Pelvic Architecture," *American Journal of Obstetrics and Gynecology* 28: 482–497.

Callon, M. (1980) "Struggles and Negotiations to Define What is Problematic and What is Not: The Sociologics of Translation," in K. Knorr, R. Krohn, R.D. Whitley (eds) *The Social Process of Scientific Investigation Yearbook 4,* Dordrecht, London and Boston, Mass.: Reidel.

—— (1986) "Some Elements of a Sociology of Translation: Domestication of the Scallops and the Fisherman of St. Brieuc Bay," in J. Law (ed.) *Power, Action, and Belief: A New Sociology of Science?,* London: Routledge & Kegan Paul.

—— (1987) "The Sociology of an Actor-network: The Case of the Electric Vehicle," in M. Callon, J. Law, A. Rip (eds) *Mapping the Dynamics of Science and Technology,* Basingstoke: Macmillan.

Callow, N.H., Callow, R.K. (1938) "The Isolation of Androsterone and Transhydroandrosterone from the Urine of Normal Women," *Biochemical Journal* 32: 1,759–1,762.

Callow, R.K., Parkes, A.S. (1936) "Production of Oestrogenic Substance by the Bird Testis", *Journal of Experimental Biology* 13: 7–11.

Canguilhem, G. (1977) *On the Normal and the Pathological,* Dordrecht: Reidel.

Capellen, D. van (1936) "Behandeling der prostatahypertrophie," *Nederlands Tijdschrift Geneeskunde* 80: 1,254–1,257.

Chatain, D. (1981) *De Pil: Pro & Contra*, Helmond: Uitgeverij Helmond.

Christian Johnson, R. (1977) "Feminism, Philanthropy and Science in the Development of the Oral Contraceptive Pill," *Pharmacy in History* 19 (2): 63–79.

Clarke, A.E. (1985) "Emergence of the Reproductive Research Enterprise: A Sociology of Biological, Medical and Agricultural Science in the United States, 1910–1940," Dissertation, University of California, San Francisco.

—— (1987a) "The Industrialization of Human Reproduction c1890–1990," Plenary Address at the Annual Conference of the U.C.-Systemwide Council of Women's Programs, U.C. Davis, California.

—— (1987b) "Research Materials and Reproductive Science in the United States, 1910–1940," in L. Gerald Geison (ed.) *Physiology in the American Context 1850–1940*, New York: American Physiological Society.

—— (1989) "A Social Worlds Research Adventure: The Case of Reproductive Science," in T. Gieryn, S. Cozzens (eds) *Theories of Science in Society*, Bloomington, Ind.: University of Indiana Press.

—— (1990a) "Women's Health Over the Life Cycle," in R. Apple (ed.) *The History of Women, Health and Medicine in America: An Encyclopedic Handbook*, New York: Garland.

—— (1990b) "Controversy and the Development of Reproductive Sciences," *Social Problems* 37: 18–37.

—— (1990c) "Changing Constellations of Interests in the American Reproductive Policy, 1900–2000", Paper presented in Washington D.C. at the American Sociological Association meeting, 1990.

—— (1993) "Embryology and the Rise of American Reproductive Science," in R. Rainger, J. Maienschein (eds) *The American Expansion of Biology*, New Brunswick, NJ: Rutgers University Press.

—— (1994) "The American Reproductive Policy Arena: Past, Present, Future," in S.B. Ruzek, V. Olessen, A. Clarke (eds) *Women's Health: Dynamics of Diversity*, Philadelphia, Pa: Temple University Press.

Collins, H.M. (1975) "The Sevens Sexes: A Study in the Sociology of a Phenomenon or the Replications of Experiments in Physics," *Sociology* 9: 205–224.

—— (1983) "The Sociology of Scientific Knowledge: Studies of Contemporary Science," *Annual Review of Sociology* 9.

Collins, H.M., Pinch, T.J. (1982) *Frames of Meaning: The Social Construction of Extraordinary Science*, London: Routledge & Kegan Paul.

Comaroff, J., Maguiri, P. (1981) "Ambiguity and the Search for Meaning: Childhood Leukemia in the Modern Clinical Context," *Social Science and Medicine* 15 B (2) 115–122.

Corner, G.W. (1965) "The Early History of Oestrogenic Hormones," *Proceedings of the Society of Endocrinology* 33: 3–18.

Council on Pharmacy and Chemistry (1939) "The Present Status of Testosterone Propionate: Three Brands, Perandren, Oreton and Neo-Hombreol (Roche-Organon) Not Acceptable for N.N.R.," *Journal of the American Medical Association* 112 (19): 1,949–1,951.

Coupland, N. (ed.) (1988) *Styles of Discourse*, London: Croom Helm.

Dale, H.H. (1935a) "Conference on the Standardisation of Sex Hormones held at London on July 30th and August 1st 1932," *Quarterly Bulletin of the Health Organisation of the League of Nations* 4: 121–128.

—— (1935b) "Report of the Second Conference on the Standardisation of Sex Hormones, held in London July 15th to 17th 1935," *Quarterly Bulletin of the Health Organisation of the League of Nations* 4: 618–630.

Diczfalusy, E. (1987) "The History of Steroidal Contraception: What is Past and

What is Present," in F. Michal (ed.) *Safety Requirements for Contraceptive Steroids: Proceedings of a Symposium on Improving Safety Requirements for Contraceptive Steroids Convened by the WHO Special Programme of Research, Development and Research Training in Human Reproduction*, Cambridge, Port Chester, Melbourne and Sydney: Cambridge University Press.

Dingemanse, E., Laqueur, E., Muhlbock, O. (1928) "Chemical Identification of Estrone in Human Male Urine," *Nature* 141: 927.

Dingemanse, E., Borchardt, A., Laqueur, E. (1937) "Capon Comb Growth-promoting Substances ("Male Hormones") in Human Urine of Males and Females of Varying Ages," *Biochemical Journal* 31: 500–507.

Doisy, A.E. (1939) "Biochemistry of the Estrogenic Compounds," in E. Allen (ed.) *Sex and Internal Secretions*, 2nd edn, Baltimore, Md: Williams & Wilkins.

—— (1972) "Isolation of a Crystalline Estrogen from Urine and the Follicular Hormone," *American Journal of Obstetrics and Gynecology* 114: 701–703.

Dongen, J.A. van (1929) "De hormoontherapie in de gynecologie," *Nederlands Tijdschrift voor Geneeskunde* 73: 3,781–3,797.

Duden, B. (1991a) "Geslecht, Biologie, Körpergeschichte. Bemerkungen zu neuer Literatur in der Körpergeschichte," *Feministische Studien* 1991 (2): 105–123.

—— (1991b) "Het maken van leven: Voortplantingstechnologie en genetische manipulatie vanuit het perspectief van een feministische wetenschapskritiek", *Tijdschrift voor Vrouwenstudies* 12 (3): 387–404.

—— (1991c) *The Woman beneath the Skin: A Doctor's Patients in Eighteenth-Century Germany*, Cambridge, Mass. and London: Harvard University Press.

Emde Boas, C. van (1933) *Nederlands Tijdschrift voor Geneeskunde* 77: 415–417.

Eng, H. (1934) "Resportion und Ausscheidung des Follikulins im menschlichen Organismus II. Mitteillung: Zur Kenntnis der Follikelausscheidung in Harn und Fezes normaler Männer," *Biochemische Zeitschrift* 274: 208–211.

Engelhardt, H.T., Caplan, A.L. (eds) (1987) *Scientific Controversies*, Cambridge: Cambridge University Press.

Esch, P. van der (1935) "Behandeling van depressies met menformon", *Nederlands Tijdschrift voor Geneeskunde* 80: 3,845–3,853.

Evans, H.M. (1939) "Endocrine Glands: Gonads, Pituitary and Adrenals," *Annual Review of Physiology*, The Hague: Martinus Nijhoff.

Fausto-Sterling, A. (1985) *Myths of Gender: Biological Theories about Women and Men*, New York: Basic Books.

—— (1993) "The Five Sexes: Why Male and Female are not enough," *The Sciences* March/April: 20–25.

Feher, M., Naddaff, R., Tazi, N. (1989) *Fragments for a History of the Human Body: Parts One, Two and Three*, New York: Zone.

Fellner, O. (1921) *Pflüger's Archiv* 189.

Fleck, L. (1979) *Genesis and Development of a Scientific Fact*, Chicago and London: University of Chicago Press.

Foucault, M. (1975) *Surveiller et punir: naissance de la prison*, Paris: Gallimard.

—— (1976) *Histoire de la sexualité, 1: La Volonté de savoir*, Paris: Gallimard.

—— (1984) *De Wil tot weten: Geschiedenis van de seksualiteit I*, Nijmegen: Socialistische Uitgeverij Nijmegen.

Fox, R.C. (1959) *Experiment Perilous: Physicians and Patients Facing the Unknown*, Glencoe, Ill.: The Free Press.

Frank, R.T. (1929) *The Female Sex Hormone*, Springfield, Ill. and Baltimore, Md: Charles C. Thomas.

—— (1931) "The Hormonal Causes of Premenstrual Tension," *Archive of Neurology and Psychiatry* 26: 1,053–1,057.

Franklin, A. (1986) *The Neglect of the Experiment*, Cambridge: Cambridge University Press.

Freud, J. (1930) "Uber Männliches (Sexual-) Hormon," *Klinische Wochenschrift* 9: 772–774.

—— (1936) "Over Geslachtshormonen," *Chemisch Weekblad* 33 (4)3: 1–14.

—— (1938) "Die Eichung der 'Männlichen' Hormonen (und ihrer Ko-Substanzen)," in E. Abderhalden (ed.) *Handbuch der biologischen Arbeitsmethoden, 1938 V Teil 3B*, Berlin and Vienna: Verlag von Urban & Schwarzenberg.

Freud, S. (1905) "Three Essays on the Theory of Sexuality," in *Sigmund Freud: The Standard Edition of the Complete Psychological Works of Sigmund Freud*, vol. 7, ed. and trans. James Strachey, in collaboration with Anna Freud, assisted by Alix Strachey and Alan Tyson, London: Hogarth Press and the Institute of Psychoanalysis.

—— (1933) *Neue Folge der Vorlesungen zur Einfuhrung in die Psychoanalyse*, Gesammelte Werke 15: 120.

Fried, B. (1982) "Boys Will Be Boys Will Be Boys: The Language of Sex and Gender," in R. Hubbard, M.S. Henefin, B. Fried (eds) *Biological Woman: The Convenient Myth*, Cambridge: Schenkman.

Galison, P. (1987) *How Experiments End*, Chicago: University of Chicago Press.

Gallagher, C., Laqueur T., (eds) (1987) *The Making of the Modern Body: Sexuality and Society in the Nineteenth Century*, Berkeley, Los Angeles and London: University of California Press.

Garcia, C.R., Pincus, G. (1964) "Clinical Considerations of Oral Hormonal Control of Human Fertility," *Clinical Obstetrics and Gynaecology* 7: 844–856.

Garcia, C.R., Pincus, G., Rock, J. (1958) "Effects of Three 19-Nor Steroids on Human Ovulation and Menstruation," *American Journal of Obstetrics and Gynecology* 166: 82–97.

Gautier, R. (1935) "The Health Organisation and Biological Standardisation," *Quarterly Bulletin of the Health Organisation* IV (3): 499–549.

Gelijns, A.C. (1991) *Innovation in Clinical Practice: The Dynamics of Medical Technology Developments*, Washington, DC: National Academy Press.

Giddens, A. (1990) *The Consequences of Modernity*, Cambridge: Polity.

Gilbert, G.N., Mulkay, M. (1984a) *Opening Pandora's Box: A Sociological Analysis of Scientific Discourse*, Cambridge: Cambridge University Press.

—— (1984b) "Experiments are the Key: Participants' Histories and Historians' Histories of Science," *Isis* 75: 105–125.

Gillespie, B., Eva, D., Johnston, R. (1979) "Carcinogenic Risk Assessment in the U.S.A. and U.K: The Case of Aldrin/Dieldrin," *Social Studies of Science* 9: 265–301.

Gooding, D., Pinch, T., Schaffer, S. (1989) *The Uses of Experiment: Studies in the Natural Sciences*, Cambridge: Cambridge University Press.

Goodman, N. (1978) *Ways of Worldmaking*, Indianapolis, Ind.: Hackett.

Gordon, L. (1976) *Woman's Body, Woman's Right: A Social History of Birth Control in America*, New York: Grossman.

Grant, E. (1986) *De bittere pil: Hoe veilig is het veiligste anticonceptiemiddel?*, Utrecht and Antwerpen: Uitgeverij Kosmos.

Greer, G. (1991) *The Change. Women, Ageing and the Menopause*, London: Hamish Hamilton.

Groenewegen, P., Berg, K. v.d., Vergragt, P. (1988) "How do Positive and Negative Images Affect Research: The Case of the Health Drug DES," Paper presented at the EASST/4S Conference in Amsterdam, November.

Gruhn, J.G., Kazer, R.R. (1989) *Hormonal Regulation of the Menstrual Cycle: The Evolution of Concepts*, New York and London: Plenum Medical.

Gupta, J.A. (1991) "Women's Bodies: The Site for the Ongoing Conquest by Reproductive Technologies," *Reproductive and Genetic Engineering* 4: 93–107.

Gustavson, R.G. (1939) "The Bioassay of Androgens and Estrogens," in E. Allen (ed.) *Sex and Internal Secretions*, 2nd edn, Baltimore, Md: Williams and Wilkins.

HAWK (1956) "30 jaar gestandariseerd oestrogeen hormoon," *Het Hormoon* 20 (5): 77–85.

Hacking, I. (1986) *Representing and Intervening: Introductory Topics in the Philosophy of Natural Science*, Cambridge: Cambridge University Press.

—— (1989) "Filosofen van het experiment," *Kennis en Methode* 13 (1): 11–27.

Hamilton, D. (1986) *The Monkey Gland Affair*, London: Chatto & Windus.

Haraway, D. (1981) "In the Beginning was the Word: The Genesis of Biological Theory," in D. Haraway *Simians, Cyborgs and Women: The Reinvention of Women*, New York: Routledge.

—— (1988) "Situated Knowledges: The Science Question in Feminism and the Privilege of Partial Perspective," *Feminist Studies* 14 (3): 575–599.

—— (1989a) *Primate Visions: Gender, Race, and Nature in the World of Modern Science*, New York and London: Routledge.

—— (1989b) "The Biopolitics of Postmodern Bodies: Determinations of Self in Immune System Discourse," *Differences* 1: 3–43.

Hardon, A. (1992) "Development of Contraceptives: General Concerns," in B. Mintzes (ed.) *A Question of Control. Women's Perspectives on the Development and Use of Contraceptive Technologies*, Report of an International Conference held in Woudschoten, The Netherlands, April 1991, Amsterdam: WEMOS Women and Pharmaceuticals Project and Health Action International.

Hardon, A., Claudio-Estrada, S. (1991) "Contraceptive Technologies, Family Planning Services, and Reproductive Rights," *VENA (Vrouwen en Autonomie Journal)* 3: 10–15.

Hartley, P. (1936) "Report on the International Biological Standards maintained at the National Institute for Medical Research, Hampstead, London, on behalf of the Health Organisation of the League of Nations," *Quarterly Bulletin of the Health Organisation of the League of Nations* 5: 713–727.

Haspels, A.A. (1985) "Hormonen en de Pil," *Cahiers Biowetenschappen en Maatschappy* 10: 19–27.

Haspels, A.A., Kremer, J. (eds) (1987) *De Pil: Een antwoord op alles wat u weten wilt over de pil*, Amsterdam: Teleboek.

Heape, W. (1913) *Sex Antagonism*, London: Constable.

Hiddinga, A. (1990) "Geordende bekkens: classificatie-systemen in de verloskunde," *Tijdschrift voor Vrouwenstudies* 11 (2): 158–175.

Hoeven, H. van der (1931) "Hormonale menstruatiestoornissen," *Nederlands Tijdschrift voor Geneeskunde* 75: 5,087–5,103.

Honegger, C. (1991) *Die Ordnung der Geslechter: Die Wissenschaften vom Menschen und das Weib*, Frankfurt and New York: Campus Verlag.

hooks, b. (1982) *Ain't I a Woman: Black Women and Feminism*, London: Pluto.

Hubbard, R. (1981) "The Emperor Doesn't Wear Any Clothes: The Impact of Feminism on Biology," in D. Spender (ed.) *Men's Studies Modified: The Impact of Feminism on the Academic Disciplines*, Oxford and New York: Pergamon.

Hubbard, R., Henifin, M.S., Fried, B. (eds) (1982) *Biological Woman: The Convenient Myth*, Cambridge, Mass.: Schenkman.

Ingle, D.W. (1971) "Gregory Goodwin Pincus," *Biographical Memoirs: National Academy of Sciences, the United States of America* 42: 229–271.

Jacobus, M., Keller, E.F., Shuttleworth, S. (eds) (1990) *Body/Politics: Women and the Discourses of Science*, New York and London: Routledge.

Jongh, S.E. de (1934a) "Menformon en zwangerschap," *Nederlands Tijdschrift voor Geneeskunde* 78: 731.

—— (1934b) "De betekenis van vrouwelijk hormoon, menformon, voor mannelijke individuen," *Nederlands Tijdschrift voor Geneeskunde* 78: 1,208–1,216.

—— (1936) ' "Vrouwelijk' en 'mannelijk' geslachtshormoon," ' *Nederlands Tijdschrift voor Geneeskunde* 80: 5,366–5,375.

—— (1937) "De beïnvloeding van het mannelijk genitaal apparaat door hormonen," *Het Hormoon* 7 (1–2): 43–49.

—— (1951) "In hoeverre verdient testosteron de naam mannelijke hormoon?," in Faculteit der Geneeskunde der Rijksuniversiteit Utrecht (ed.) *De moderne aspecten der endocrinologie: speciaal der praktische hormonologie*, Amsterdam: Scheltema en Holkema's Boekhandel en Uitgeverijmaatschappij.

Jongh, S.E. de, Laqueur, E., Dingemanse, E. (1929) "Over vrouwelijk hormoon (menformon) in mannelijke organismen; iets over het begrip specificiteit," *Nederlands Tijdschrift Geneeskunde*. 73: 771–75.

Jordanova, L. (1980) "Natural Facts: A Historical Perspective on Science and Sexuality," in C. MacCormack, and M. Strathern (eds) *Nature, Culture and Gender*, New York: Cambridge University Press.

—— (1989) *Sexual Visions: Images of Gender in Science and Medicine between the Eighteenth and Twentieth Centuries*, New York and London: Harvester Wheatsheaf.

Kaufert, P.A., McKinlay, S.M. (1987) "Estrogen-replacement Therapy: The Production of Medical Knowledge and the Emergence of Policy," in E. Lewin, V. Olesen (eds) *Women, Health and Healing*, New York and London: Tavistock.

Keller, E. Fox (1982) "Feminism and Science," *Signs: Journal of Women in Culture and Society* 7 (1): 589–595

—— (1984) *Reflections on Gender and Science*, New Haven, Conn.: Yale University Press.

Klein, M., Parkes, A. (1937) "The Progesteron-like Action of Testosterone and Certain Related Compounds," *Proceedings of the Royal Society London* 3: 574–579.

Knoke, D., Kuklinsky, J.H. (1982) *Network Analysis*, Beverly Hills, Calif.: Sage.

Knorr-Cetina, K.D. (1981a) *The Manufacture of Knowledge: An Essay on the Constructivist and Contextual Nature of Science*, Oxford: Pergamon.

—— (1981b) "The Micro-Sociological Challenge of Macro-Sociology: Towards a Reconstruction of Social Theory and Methodology," in K. Knorr-Cetina, A.V. Cicourel (eds) *Advances in Social Theory and Methodology: Toward an Integration of Micro and Macro-Sociologies*, Boston, Mass.: Routledge & Kegan Paul.

—— (1983) "The Ethnographic Study of Scientific Work: Towards a Constructivist Interpretation of Science," in K. Knorr-Cetina (ed.) *Science Observed: Perspectives on the Social Studies of Science*, London: Sage.

Koch, F.C. (1936) "The Biochemistry and Physiological Significance of the Male Sex Hormone," *Journal of Urology* 35: 383–390.

—— (1939) "The Biochemistry of Androgens," in E. Allen (ed.) *Sex and Internal Secretions*, 2nd edn, Baltimore, Md: Williams & Wilkins.

Kochakian, Ch.D. (1938) "Excretion and Fate of Androgens: Conversion of Androgens to Estrogens," *Endocrinology* 23: 463–467.

Kohaus-Altmeyer, C. (1981) "Die Verhütung der Männerpille," *Emma* 3: 6–8.

Kohler, R.E. (1982) *From Medical Chemistry to Biochemistry: The Making of a Biomedical Discipline*, Cambridge and New York: Cambridge University Press.

Kohler Riessman, C. (1983) "Women and Medicalization: A New Perspective," *Social Policy* 14: 13–19.

Korenchevsky, Vl., Hall, K. (1938) "Manifold Effects of Male and Female Sex Hormones in Both Sexes," *Nature* 142: 998.

Korenchevsky, Vl., Dennison, M., Hall, K. (1937) "The Action of Testosterone Propionate on Normal Adult Female Rats," *Biochemical Journal* 31: 780–785.

Kruif, P. de (undated) *Het Mannelijk Hormoon*, Nederlandse bewerking door C.C. Bender, Uitgeverij Keesing, Amsterdam.

Kuhn, T. (1970) *The Structure of Scientific Revolutions*, 2nd edn, Chicago: University of Chicago Press.

Laqueur, E. (1935) "Sexualhormone und Prostratahypertrophie," Unpublished lecture, Organon's Archive on the correspondence between Ernst Laqueur and Organon. Lecture dated 9 November.

—— (1937) "Orgaan en hormoon therapie," *Het Hormoon* 7 (1–2): 5–7.

Laqueur, E., Hart, P.C., Jongh, S.E. de (1927a) "Over een vrouwelijk geslachtshormoon (menformon)," *Nederlands Tijdschrift voor Geneeskunde* 71: 2,077–2,089.

Laqueur, E., Dingemanse, E., Hart, P.C., Jong, S.E. de (1927b) "Female Sex Hormone in Urine of Men," *Klinische Wochenschrift* 6: 1,859.

Laqueur, T. (1990) *Making Sex: Body and Gender from the Greeks to Freud*, Cambridge, Mass. and London: Harvard University Press.

Latour, B. (1987) *Science in Action: How to Follow Scientists and Engineers through Society*, Milton Keynes: Open University Press.

—— (1988) *The Pasteurization of France*, Cambridge, Mass. and London: Harvard University Press.

Latour, B., Woolgar, S. (1979) *Laboratory Life: The Social Construction of Scientific Facts*, Beverly Hills, Calif. and London: Sage.

Lauretis, T. de (1984) *Alice Doesn't*, Bloomington, Ind.: Indiana University Press.

Leichner, P., Harper, D. (1982) "Sex Role Ideology among Physicians," *CMA Journal* 27.

Lewin, M. (1984) "Rather Worse than Folly? Psychology Measures Femininity and Masculinity 1," in M. Lewin (ed.) *In the Shadow of the Past: Psychology Portrays the Sexes*, New York: Columbia University Press.

Lichtenstern, R. (1920) "Bisherige Erfolge der Hodentransplantation beim Menschen," *Jahreskurse fur artzliche Fortbildung* 11 (4): 8–11.

Liebenau, J. (1987) *Medical Science and Medical Industry: The Formation of the American Pharmaceutical Industry*, London: Macmillan Press, in association with Business History Unit, University of London.

Lillie, F.R. (1939) "Biological Introduction," in E. Allen (ed.) *Sex and Internal Secretions*, 2nd edn, Baltimore, M.D: Williams & Wilkins.

Liskin, L., Rinehart, W., Blackburn, R., Rutledge, A.H. (1985) "Female Sterilization," *Population Reports* 9: 128–129.

Long Hall, D. (1975) "Biology, Sexism and Sex Hormones in the 1920s," in M. Wartofsky, C. Could (eds) *Women and Philosophy*, New York: Putnam.

—— (1976) "The Social Implications of the Scientific Study of Sex," *The Scholar and the Feminist* IV, New York: The Women's Center of Barnard College: 11–21.

Long, D. (1987) "The Physiological Identity of American Sex Researchers," in G. L. Geison (ed.) *Physiology in the American Context 1850–1940*, Bethesda, Md: American Physiological Society.

—— (1990) "Moving Reprints: A Historian Looks at Sex Research Publications of the 1930s," *Journal of the History of Medicine and Allied Sciences*, 45, (3): 452–468.

Longino H. (1990) *Science as Social Knowledge: Values and Objectivity in Scientific Inquiry*, Princeton, NJ and Oxford: Princeton University Press.

Longino, H., Doell, R. (1983) "Body, Bias, and Behavior: A Comparative Analysis of Reasoning in Two Areas of Biological Science," *Signs: Journal of Women in Culture and Society* 9, (2): 207–227.

Lynch, M. (1985) *Art and Artifact in Laboratory Science: A Study of Shop Work and Shop Talk in a Research Laboratory*, London: Routledge & Kegan Paul.

McClung, I. (1902) "The Role of Chromosomal Factor in Sex Determination," *Biological Bulletin* 3 (1–2): 43–84.

McLaughlin, L. (1982) *The Pill, John Rock and the Church: The Biography of a Revolution*, Boston, Mass. and Toronto: Little, Brown.

Maisel, A.Q. (1965) *The Hormone Quest*, New York: Random House.

Marks, H.M. (1987a) "Notes from the Underground: The Social Organisation of Therapeutic Research," in D. Long, R. Maulits (eds) *Grand Rounds: 100 Years of Internal Medicine*, Philadelphia, Pa: University of Pennsylvania Press

—— (1987b) "Ideas and Reforms: Therapeutic Experiments and Medical Practice, 1900–1980," Thesis, Massaschusetts Institute of Technology, Cambridge, Mass.

Marsden, P.V., Lin, N. (1981) *Social Structure and Network Analysis*, Beverly Hills, Calif.: Sage.

Martin, E. (1987) *The Woman in the Body. A Cultural Analysis of Reproduction*, Boston, Mass.: Beacon.

Mead, M. (1950) *Sex and Temperament in Three Primitive Societies*, New York: New American Library (Mentor Books).

Medvei, V.C. (1983) *A History of Endocrinology*, The Hague: MTP Press.

Messent, P.R. (1976) "Female Hormones and Behaviour," in B. Lloyd, J. Archer (eds) *Exploring Sex Differences*, London and New York: Academic Press.

Meyer-Bahlburg, H.F.L. (1977) "Sex Hormones and Male Homosexuality in Comparative Perspective," *Archives Sexual Behavior* 297–326.

—— (1984) "Psychoendocrine Research on Sexual Orientation, Current Status and Future Options," *Progress in Brain Research* 61: 375–399.

Mintzes, B. (ed.) (1992) *A Question of Control: Women's Perspectives on the Development and Use of Contraceptive Technologies*, Report of an International Conference held in Woudschoten, The Netherlands, April 1991, *Amsterdam: WEMOS Women and Pharmaceuticals Project and Health Action International.*

Mol, A. (1988) "Baarmoeders, pigment en pyramiden," *Tijdschrift voor Vrouwenstudies* 9 (3): 276–90.

Mol, A., Lieshout, P. (1989) *Ziek is het woord niet: Medicalisering, normalisering en de veranderende taal van huisartsgeneeskunde en geestelijke gezondheidszorg 1945–1985*, Nijmegen: SUN (Socialistische Uitgeverij Nijmegen).

Money, J. (1980) "History of Concepts of Determination," in J. Money, *Love and Lovesickness: The Science of Sex, Gender Difference and Pairbonding*, Baltimore, Md and London: Johns Hopkins University Press.

Money, J., Ehrhardt, A. (1972) *Man and Woman, Boy and Girl*, Baltimore, Md: Johns Hopkins University Press.

Moore, C.R., Price, D. (1932) "Gonad Hormone Functions: Reciprocal Influence between Gonads and Hypophysis with its Bearing on Problems of Sex Hormone Antagonism," *American Journal of Anatomy* 50: 13–71.

Morawski, J.G. (1987) "The Troubled Quest for Masculinity, Femininity, and Androgyny," in P. Shaver, C. Hendrick (eds) *Sex and Gender*, Beverly Hills, London and New Delhi: Sage..

Niemi, S. (1987) "Andrology as a Speciality: Its Origin," *Journal of Andrology* 8: 201–203.

Novak, E. (1939) "Clinical Employment of the Female Sex Hormones," *Endocrinology* 25: 423–428.

Oakley, A. (1972) *Sex, Gender and Society*, London: Temple Smith.

Organon Archive on the Correspondence of Ernst Laqueur with Organon Employees, 1923–1940.

Oudshoorn, N. (1994) "Female or Male: The Classification of Homosexuality and Gender," *Journal of Homosexuality* 27 (3–4).

Outshoorn, J. (1979) "Vrouwenbeweging, seksualiteit en geboorteregeling in Nederland 1880–1979," *Socialisties-Feministiese Teksten* 3: 60–73.

Overbeek, G.A., Visser, J. de (1956) "A New Substance with Progestational Activity," *Acta Endocrinologica* 22: 318–329.

Paglia, C. (1991) *Sexual Personae: Art and Decadence from Nefertiti to Emily Dickinson*, Harmondsworth: Penguin.

Parkes, A.S. (1938) "Terminology of Sex Hormones," *Nature* 141: 12.

—— (1937) "Androgenic Activity of Ovarian Extracts," *Nature* 139: 965.

—— (1938) "Ambisexual Activity of the Gonads," in *Les Hormonnes sexuelles*, Paris: Colloque International Fondation Singer-Polignac.

—— (1966) "The Rise of Reproductive Endocrinology 1926–1940," *Proceedings of the Society of Endocrinology* 34 (3): 20–32.

—— (1985) *Off Beat Biologist: The Autobiography of Alan S. Parkes*, Cambridge: Galton Foundation.

Pasveer, B. (1992) "Shadows of Knowledge: Making a Representing Practice in Medicine – X-ray Pictures and Pulmonary Tuberculosis, 1895–1930," PhD thesis, University of Amsterdam.

Petterson, W. (1933) "Kritisches zur paradoxen Keimdrusen Therapie," *Fortschriftte der Therapie* 9: 711–718.

Pinch, T. (1985) "Towards an Analysis of Scientific Observation: The Externality and Evidential Significance of Observational Reports in Physics," *Social Studies of Science* 15: 3–36.

—— (1993) "Testing 'One, Two, Three . . . Testing!' Toward a Sociology of Testing," *Science, Technology and Human Values* 18 (1): 25–41.

Pinch, T.J., Bijker, W.E. (1987) "The Social Construction of Facts and Artefacts or How the Sociology of Science and the Sociology of Technology Might Benefit Each Other," in W.E. Bijker, T.P. Hughes, T.J. Pinch (eds) *The Social Construction of Technological Systems: New Directions in the Sociology and History of Technology*, Cambridge, Mass.: MIT Press.

Pincus, G. (1958) "Fertility Control with Oral Medication," *American Journal of Obstetrics and Gynecology* 75: 1,333–1,347.

—— (1959) "Progestational Agents and the Control of Fertility," *Vitamins and Hormones* 169: 307–325.

—— (1965) *The Control of Fertility*, New York and London: Academic Press.

Pincus, G., Chang, M.C., Hafez, E.S.E., Zarrow, M.X., Merrill, A. (1956) "Effects of Certain 19-Nor Steroids on Reproductive Processes in Animals," *Science* 124: 890–891.

Pincus, G., Garcia, C.R., Rock, J., Paniagua, M., Pendleton, A., Larague, F., Nicola, R., Borno, R., Rean, V. (1959) "Effectiveness of a Progestine-estrogen Combination upon Fertility, Menstrual Phenomena, and Health," *Science* 130: 81–83.

Pincus, G., Garcia, C.R., Paniague, M., Shepard, J. (1962) "Ethynodiol Diacetate as a New Highly Potent Oral Inhibitor of Ovulation," *Science* 138: 439–440.

Pinkhof, H. (1927a) "Kwakzalverijreclame in tramwagens," *Nederlands Tijdschrift voor Geneeskunde* 71: 213–215.

—— (1927b) "De geneesmiddelen anarchie," *Nederlands Tijdschrift Geneeskunde*. 72: 2,551–2,552.

—— (1928) "De economische betekenis der menstruatie," *Nederlands Tijdschrift voor Geneeskunde* 73: 1,948.

—— (1931) "Onvruchtbaar maken door middel van een hormoon," *Nederlands Tijdschrift voor Geneeskunde* 75: 99.

Piotrow, P.T. (1973) *World Population Crisis: The United States Response*, New York, Washington and London: Praeger.

Pollock, S. (1984) "Refusing to Take Women Seriously: Side Effects and the Politics of Contraception," in R. Arditti (ed.) *Test Tube Women: What Future for Motherhood?*, London: Pandora.

Pomata, G. (1983) "La Storia delle Donna: una questione di confine," *Il mondo contemporaineo* 10. Dutch translation, Pomata, G. (1987) "De geschiedenis van vrouwen: een kwestie van grenzen," *Socialisties-Feministiese Teksten* 10: 61–113.

Pratt, J. P. (1939) "Sex Functions in Man," in E. Allen (ed.) *Sex and Internal Secretions*, Baltimore, Md: Williams & Wilkins.

Price, D. (1975) "Feedback Control of Gonadal and Hypophyseal Hormones: Evolution of the Concept," in J. Meites, B.M. McCann (eds) *Pioneers in Neuro-endocrinology*, New York and London: Plenum.

Ramirez de Arellano, A.B., Seipp, C. (1983) *Colonialism, Catholicism, and Contraception: A History of Birth Control in Puerto Rico*, Chapel Hill, NC and London: University of North Carolina Press.

Reed, J. (1984) *The Birth Control Movement and American Society: From Private Vice to Public Virtue*, Princeton, NJ: Princeton University Press.

Richards, E. (1988) "The Politics of Therapeutic Evaluation: The Vitamin C and Cancer Controversy," *Social Studies of Science* 18: 653–701.

Rock, J. (1963) *The Time has Come: A Catholic Doctor's Proposals to End the Battle over Birth Control*, New York: Alfred A. Knopf.

Rock, J., Pincus, G. (1956) "Effects of Certain 19-Nor Steroids on the Normal Human Menstrual Cycle," *Science* 124: 891–893.

Rock, J., Garcia, C.R., Pincus, G. (1957) "Synthetic Progestins in the Normal Human Menstrual Cycle," *Recent Progress in Hormone Research* 13: 323–346.

Rogers, L. (1976) "Male Hormones and Behaviour," in B. Lloyd, J. Archer (eds) *Exploring Sex Differences*, London and New York: Academic Press.

Rubin, G. (1975) "The Traffic in Women. Notes on the Political Economy of Sex," in G. Rubin (ed.) *Toward an Anthropology of Women*, New York: Monthly Review Press.

Santgiorgi, P. (1937) "Androstine in disease of women," *Rassegna internazionale di clinica en terapeutica* 18: 871–874.

Sayers, J. (1982) *Biological Politics: Feminist and Anti-Feminist Perspectives*, New York: Tavistock.

Schaffer, S. (1990) "A Manufactory of Ohms: The Integrity of Victorian Values," Unpublished lecture held at the Science Dynamics Department, University of Amsterdam, November.

Schiebinger, L. (1986) "Skeletons in the Closet: The First Illustrations of the Female Skeleton in the nineteenth-century Anatomy," *Representations* 14: 42–83.

—— (1989) *The Mind has No Sex? Women in the Origins of Modern Science.* Cambridge, Mass. and London: Harvard University Press.

Schmidt, G. (1984) "Allies and Persecutors: Science and Medicine in the Homosexuality Issues," *Journal of Homosexuality* 10 (3/4): 127–140.

Schoon, L. (1990) *In de Greep van de Gynecoloog*, Amsterdam: Pieter Lakeman.

Seaman, B. (1969) *The Doctor's Case against the Pill*, New York: Peter H. Wyden.

Seaman, B., Seaman, G. (19778) *Women and the Crisis in Sex Hormones. An Investigation of the Dangerous Uses of Hormones: from Birth Control to Menopause and the Safe Alternatives*, Brighton, Sussex: Harvester.

Segal, S.J., Atkinson, L.E. (1973) "Biological Effects of Oral Contraceptive Steroids," in R.O. Greep, E.B. Atwood (eds) *Handbook of Physiology: A Critical Comprehensive Presentation of Physiological Knowledge and Concepts*, Washington, DC: American Physiological Society.

Shapin, S., Schaffer, S. (1985) *Leviathan and the Air Pump: Hobbes, Boyle and the Experimental Life*, Princeton, NJ: Princeton University Press.

Shaver, P., Hendrick, C. (eds) (1987) *Sex and Gender*, Beverly Hills, London and New Delhi: Sage.

Siebke, H. (1931) "Presence of Androkinin in Female Organism," *Archiv für Gynaekologie.* 146: 417–462.

Smart, B. (1992) *Modern Conditions, Postmodern Controversies*, London and New York: Routledge.

Sneader, W. (1985) *Drug Discovery: The Evolution of Modern Medicines*, Chichesters, New York, Brisbane, Toronto and Singapore: John Wiley.

Snoo, K. de (1940) "De gynecologie en de moderne vrouw," *Nederlands Tijdschrift voor Geneeskunde* 84: 3,940–3,946.

Star, S.L. (1989) *Regions of the Mind: Brain Research and the Quest for Scientific Certainty*, Stanford, Calif.: University of Stanford Press.

Starling, E.H. (1905) "The Croonian Lectures on the Chemical Correlation of the Functions of the Body," *Lancet* ii: 339–41.

Starr, P. (1982) *The Social Transformation of American Medicine*, New York: Basic Books.

Steinach, E. (1916) "Pubertats druesen und Zwitterbildung," *Archiv für Entwicklungsdynamik* 42: 307–332.

—— (1926) "Antagonische Wirkungen der Keimdrusen Hormone," *Biologia Generalis* 2: 815–834.

Strachey, J. (ed.) (1965) *The New Introductory Letters on Psychoanalysis*, New York and London: W.W. Norton.

Stycos, J.M. (1962) "Experiments in Social Change: The Caribbean, Fertility Studies," in C.V. Kiser (ed.) *Research in Family Planning*, Princeton, NJ: Princeton University Press.

Swann, J.P. (1988) *Academic Scientists and the Pharmaceutical Industry*, Baltimore, MD and London: Johns Hopkins University Press.

Tausk, M. (1931) "Over de hormonale zwangerschapsreaktie," *Het Hormoon* 1 (2): 13–16.

—— (1932a) "Over een mannelijke geslachtshormoon," *Het Hormoon* 1 (7): 49–54.

—— (1932b) "Over de doosering van ovariaalhormoon (menformon) in de praktijk," *Het Hormoon* 2 (2): 15–17.

—— (1933) "De hormonale behandeling van de zogenaamde hypertrophie van de prostata," *Het Hormoon* 2 (8): 71–73.

—— (1934a) "De beteekenis van de vrouwelijke geslachtshormonen (menformon en progesterine) in het bijzonder gedurende de zwangerschap," *Het Hormoon* 3 (6): 41–45.

—— (1934b) "Over de hormonale behandeling der stoornissen van het mannelijk geslachtsapparaat," *Het Hormoon* 4 (4): 25–29.

—— (1934c) "Iets over het verband tussen het endocrine systeem en gezwelvorming," *Het Hormoon* 3 (7): 49–57.

—— (1935) "In het vijfde jaar," *Het Hormoon* 5 (1): 1.

—— (1937) "Orgaan en hormoontherapie," *Het Hormoon* 7 (1): 6.

—— (1938a) "Uitscheiding van hormonen in de urine van normale mensen", *Het Hormoon* 7 (5): 89–97.

—— (1938b) "Over de toepassing van esters van testosteron," *Het Hormoon* 7, (10): 131–136.

—— (1939a) "Over de invloed van het mannelijke hormoon, testoron, op het vrouwelijke organisme," *Het Hormoon* 8 (10): 145–152.

—— (1939b) "Oestrogene stoffen en gezwelvorming," *Het Hormoon* 8 (7): 121–131.

—— (1948) Editorial introduction *Het Hormoon* 13 (1): 1–3.

—— (1978) *Organon: De geschiedenis van een bijzondere Nederlandse Onderneming*, Nijmegen: Dekker en Van de Vegt.

Temin, P. (1980) *Taking Your Medicine: Drug Regulation in the United States*, Cambridge, Mass. and London: Harvard University Press.

Thomson, J. A. (1914) "Review of *Sex Antagonism*," *Nature* 93: 346.

Toulouse, E., Schiff, P., Simmonnet, H. (1935) "Search for Female Sex Hormones in Urine of Men with Psychosexual Disturbances", *Annual of Medical Psychology* 93: 440–446.

Travis, G.D.L. (1981) "Replicating Replication? Aspects of Social Construction of Learning in Planarian Worms," *Social Studies of Science* 11: 11–32.

Treichler, P.A. (1990) "Feminism, Medicine, and the Meaning of Childbirth," in M. Jacobus, E.F. Keller, S. Shuttleworth (eds) *Body/Politics: Women and the Discourses of Science*, New York and London: Routledge.

Tschopp, E. (1935) "Die Physiologischen Wirkingen des Kunstlichen Männlichen Sexual Hormons," *Klinische Wochenschrift* 14: 1,064–1,068.

Tyler, E.T., Olson, H.J. (1959) "Fertility Promoting and Inhibiting Effects of New Steroid Hormonal Substances," *Journal of the American Medical Association* 169: 1,843–1,855.

Vaughan, P. (1972) *The Pill on Trial*, Harmondsworth: Penguin.

Veatch, R.M. (1981) "Federal Regulation of Medicine and Biomedical Research: Power, Authority and Legitimacy" in S.F. Spicker, J.M. Healy, H.T. Engelhardt (eds) *The Law–Medicine Relation*, Dordrecht: Reidel: 75–91.

Verbrugge, L., Steiner, R.P. (1981) "Physician Treatment of Men and Women Patients: Sex Bias or Appropriate Care?" *Medical Care* 19: 609–632.

Vos, R. (1989) *Drugs Looking for Diseases: A Descriptive Model for the Process of Innovative Drug Research with Special Reference to the Development of the Beta Blockers and the Calcium Antagonists*, Proefschrift Rijksuniversiteit Groningen.

Vries, G. de, Boon, L. (1986) "Een intellectuele zeppelin en zijn bemanning," *Kennis en Methode* 1: 28–46.

Walsh, J. (1985) "The Scientific Work of Guy Marrian (1904–1981) Mainly with Respect to Steroid Hormones," Library-based Dissertation, University of Oxford.

Ward, M.C. (1986) *Poor Women and Powerful Men. America's Great Experiment in Family Planning*, Boulder, Colo. and London: Westview Press.

Warren, F.L. (1935) "Alleged Oestrogenic Activity of the Male Sex Hormone," *Nature* 135: 234.

Werthessen, N.T., Johnson, R.C. (1974) "Pincogenesis: Pathenogenesis in Rabbits by Gregory Pincus," *Biology and Medicine* 18: 86–94.

Whalen, R.E. (1984) "Multiple Actions of Steroids and their Antagonists," *Archives of Sexual Behavior* 13: 497- 501.

Whitley, R.D. (1974) "Cognitive and Social Institutionalization of Scientific Specialties and Research Areas," *Social Processes of Scientific Development*, London and Boston, Mass.: Routledge & Kegan Paul.

Wijngaard, M. van den (1991a) "Acceptance of Scientific Theories and Images of Masculinity and Feminity," *Journal of the History of Biology* 24 (1): 19–49.

—— (1991b) "Reinventing the Sexes: Feminism and Biomedical Construction of Femininity and Masculinity 1959–1985," Thesis, University of Amsterdam.

Wolffers, I., Hardon, A., Janssen, J. (1989) *Marketing Fertility: Women, Menstruation and the Pharmaceutical Industry*, Amsterdam: Wemos.

Woolgar, S. (1991) "Configuring the User: the Case of Usability Trials," in J. Law (ed.) *A Sociology of Monsters: Essays on Power, Technology and Domination*, London: Routledge.

Wright, C.A. (1938) "Further Studies of Endocrine Aspects of Homosexuality," *Medical Records*, 18 May: 449–452.

Zondek, B. (1930) "Ueber die Hormone des Hypophysenvorderlappens," *Klinische Wochenschrift* 9.

—— (1934a) "Mass Excretion of Oestrogenic Hormone in the Urine of the Stallion," *Nature* 133: 209–210.

—— (1934b) "Oestrogenic Hormone in the Urine of the Stallion," *Nature* 133 494.
Zondek, B., Finkelstein, M. (1966) "Professor Bernard Zondek: An Interview," *Journal of Reproductive Fertility* 12: 3–19.

Index

Note: Numbers in italics denote illustrations